The *Best Friends* Book of
Alzheimer's Activities

Additional titles available
on *Best Friends*™ care practices:

The Best Friends Approach to Alzheimer's Care
by Virginia Bell & David Troxel

The Best Friends Staff:
Building a Culture of Care in Alzheimer's Programs
by Virginia Bell & David Troxel

Best Friends (VHS video)
produced by the Lexington/Bluegrass Alzheimer's Association

To order, contact Health Professions Press, Inc.
Post Office Box 10624 • Baltimore, MD 21285-0624
1-888-337-8808 • http://www.healthpropress.com

For additional information on the Best Friends™ approach,
visit **www.bestfriendsapproach.com**

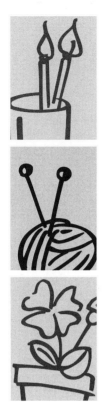

The *Best Friends* Book of
Alzheimer's Activities

Volume One

147 fun, easy, and enriching activities

Virginia Bell, M.S.W.

David Troxel, M.P.H.

Tonya M. Cox, M.S.W.

Robin Hamon, M.S.W.

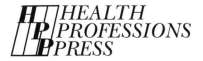

HEALTH
PROFESSIONS
PRESS

Baltimore • London • Sydney

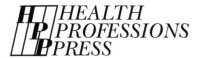

Health Professions Press
Post Office Box 10624
Baltimore, MD 21285-0624

www.healthpropress.com

First printing, September 2004.
Second printing, October 2005.

Typeset by Erin Geoghegan.
Manufactured in the United States of America by
Versa Press, East Peoria, Illinois.

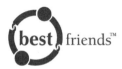

Best Friends™ is a trademark of Health Professions Press, Inc.

The following *Best Friends*™ titles are also available from Health Professions Press, Inc.:

> *The Best Friends Approach to Alzheimer's Care*
>
> *The Best Friends Staff: Building a Culture of Care in Alzheimer's Programs*
>
> *Best Friends* (VHS video)
>
> Incentives, such as t-shirts for staff, are also available.

To order, contact Health Professions Press, Inc., Post Office Box 10624, Baltimore, MD 21285-0624 (1-888-337-8808; http://www.healthpropress.com)

For more information about the Best Friends™ approach, visit www.bestfriendsapproach.com.

Library of Congress Cataloging-in-Publication Data
The best friends book of Alzheimer's activities/ Virginia Bell ... [et al.].
   p.   cm.
ISBN-13: 978-1-878812-88-9 (papercover: alk. Paper)
ISBN-10: 1-878812-88-2 (papercover: alk. Paper)
  1. Alzheimer's disease—Patients—Rehabilitation.   2. Alzheimer's disease—Patients—Long-term care.
3. Occupational therapy.   4. Recreational therapy.   I. Bell, Virginia
RC523.B47 2004
  362.196'831—dc22   2004009606

British Library Cataloguing in Publication data are available from the British Library.

Contents

About the Authors

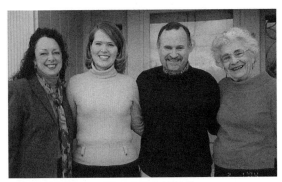

Left to right: R.Hamon, T.Cox, D.Troxel, V.Bell

Virginia Bell, M.S.W., is Program Consultant for the Greater Kentucky/Southern Indiana Chapter of the Alzheimer's Association. She is the founder of that association's Best Friends Center, an adult dementia-specific day center formerly known as the Helping Hand Day Program. With David Troxel, she has co-authored numerous articles on dementia care and three books. She has lectured about the Best Friends approach in more than 20 countries. She can be reached at vbellky@aol.com.

David Troxel, M.P.H., most recently served as the President and CEO of the California Central Coast Alzheimer's Association, Santa Barbara, California. Today he is a consultant and speaker for dementia care and long-term care programs. He has worked in the field of dementia care since 1986 and currently serves on the Ethics Advisory Panel of the national Alzheimer's Association. With Virginia Bell, he has co-authored numerous articles on dementia care and three books. He can be reached at sbdavidt@aol.com.

Tonya M. Cox, M.S.W., is Vice President of Education and Programs for the Alzheimer's Association serving greater Kentucky and southern Indiana. She began working in dementia care in 1995 in The Best Friends Center developing and leading activities for persons with memory loss. She also teaches and presents on activity programming and caring for persons with dementia. She can be reached at tonya.cox@alz.org.

Robin Hamon, M.S.W., is Family Support Coordinator for the Alzheimer's Disease Research Center at the University of Kentucky Sanders Brown Center on Aging. She worked with the Lexington-Bluegrass chapter of the Alzheimer's Association for 11 years. During her tenure as program manager for The Best Friends Center, she developed a creative art training program for staff and volunteers working with persons with dementia. Her special interests are in training and providing creative arts experiences for *persons* with dementia. She can be reached at Robin.Hamon@uky.edu.

Activities and the Best Friends Approach to Alzheimer's Care

A young man working as an activity director in an assisted living community in California recently spoke at a conference and expressed frustration about his work. "I follow the recipes in the activity books, I try to throw my own ideas in, I do all the arts and crafts stuff, but I'm in a rut. The programs are falling flat. I feel like I'm on the softball field, playing for my team, but always striking out!" The purpose of this book is to help individuals such as the young activity director rethink and retool their activity programs. It *is* possible to find the "sweet spot" and hit a home run when it comes to activities.

The Best Friends Book of Alzheimer's Activities is written for family caregivers, staff, and volunteers looking for creative and meaningful ways to plan and implement activities for *persons* with Alzheimer's disease and related dementias. The book is based on the Best Friends™ model of Alzheimer's care, a model developed by Virginia Bell and David Troxel in 1996 that is now in use around the world. The philosophy of the Best Friends model, simply put, is that what *persons* with Alzheimer's disease need most is a friend, a "best friend," who will provide loving care, accept their illness, and learn what we call the "knack" of caregiving.

The Best Friends approach to Alzheimer's care helps family and professional caregivers recast or rethink their own life and work with *persons* with dementia. It can turn the daily stress and challenges of caregiving into a more rewarding and successful experience.

ABOUT THE BEST FRIENDS MODEL

The Best Friends model is based upon the following principles:

Understanding what it is like to have Alzheimer's disease or related dementias—Best Friends understand that behaviors that seem strange or unreasonable become quite understandable when you know their origins. The Best Friends approach suggests that knowing the cause of a behavior allows you to give people what they need, when they need it, whether it's reassurance, physical contact, or a comment or gesture that helps them "save face."

Learning the basics of dementia—Best Friends do not need to become experts at research, but it is important to have a good understanding of the basics of Alzheimer's disease and other related dementias. This helps staff members accept sometimes-puzzling behaviors. It also helps staff spot treatable illnesses or conditions that affect daily life and a *person's* ability to participate in activities. This book is not written to discuss the diagnosis, treatment, and research issues surrounding dementia; we assume some basic knowledge. If you want more information about Alzheimer's disease we encourage you to check out reputable web sites and some of the books and sources mentioned in the Resources section (see page 197).

Strength-based assessment—Best Friends focus on what a *person* can still do, instead of the things a *person* with dementia can no longer do. Does the *person* enjoy music, reading the newspaper, or taking walks? Don't aim too low with your activity programming—this robs a *person* of dignity. If you aim too high, however, you'll invite frustration and failure.

Knowing the person's life story well—Best Friends learn as much as they can about the life stories, traditions, and values of *person*s in their care. This instantly helps personalize an activity because you can link the activity to a past or present interest and ability of the participant. Readers will note that each activity discusses the life story and how it can be used to give the activity more value.

Effective communication—Best Friends communicate well and know the "dos" and "don'ts" of communication with *person*s with dementia. Practicing active listening, speaking clearly and with simple sentences, giving compliments, and asking opinions help us better connect to *person*s with dementia and build a successful activity program. Each activity in this book includes "conversation starters" that will be useful for caregivers looking for ways to get the most out of an activity.

Recasting relationships—The Best Friends model encourages caregivers to rethink their relationship with *person*s in their care from "resident" or "client" to friend. Doing this allows relationships to form and makes possible activities that enrich the lives of everyone. Recasting relationships also works in home-based care settings, whether a paid worker or a family member is providing care.

For more information about the Best Friends model, we refer you to this book's companion volumes, *The Best Friends Approach to Alzheimer's Care* (Health Professions Press, 1996) or *The Best Friends Staff: Building a Culture of Care in Alzheimer's Programs* (Health Professions Press, 2001). A book for family caregivers was published in 2002 called *A Dignified Life* (Health Communications, Inc., 2002).

Developing Knack

As you rethink or recast your relationship to the *person* with dementia, you will gradually develop what we call "the knack." Knack is an old-fashioned word with a meaning that is relevant for quality Alzheimer's care. It means "the art of doing difficult things with ease" or "clever tricks and strategies." It is the goal or ultimate outcome of the Best Friends model.

When you follow the activities in the book, you take an everyday activity and add extra value and pizzazz. You can turn a meal into an opportunity for sharing life stories, a walk into a time to explore nature, brushing teeth into an opportunity to tell a joke, and an art activity into one that touches the spirit. A benefit of this book is that a staff or family member who follows the suggestions listed with each activity will gradually learn tricks and strategies to employ in almost any setting! They will develop knack!

In writing this book, we spent time talking with individuals who have early-stage Alzheimer's disease (or a related dementia). They consistently said that they value creative activities as a tool for maintaining quality of life. Their voices echo through much of this book as does the authors' optimism that there will someday be an effective treatment or cure for Alzheimer's disease.

Activity Principles

Here are some principles of activity programming done the Best Friends way that form the foundation of this book.

The Art Is Not in What Is Done, It's in the Doing—The process of the activity is always more important than the result or end product. The activity involving handmade bird feeders (see page 79) is a good example. Enjoy the process of the activity. It doesn't matter if the feeder fits together exactly or has a perfect paint job.

Activities Should Tap into Past Interests and Skills—Consider the unique life story each of us has when thinking about activities. The home-based activity around laundry (see page 173), for example, would be different for a *person* with dementia who did laundry the minute a shirt hit the floor versus someone who did not mind wearing the same shirt several times before washing it.

Activities Should Be Adult in Nature—Activities that are unnecessarily juvenile can provoke frustration, anger, or apathy. The *person* with dementia can sense when an activity is demeaning or obviously busy work. Some *persons* respond positively to dolls and children's toys, but you should not use this as an excuse to keep all activities at this level. Good examples of adult activities appear throughout the book.

Activities Should Recall a Person's *Work-Related Past*—Work plays a major role in many of our lives and many of us have a need to be productive and valued. The activity revolving around money (see page 148) will have a different flavor depending on the past occupation of the *person* with dementia and whether he or she dealt with finance.

Activities Should Stimulate the Senses—Although some of the senses diminish with age, many remain strong. Most successful activities stimulate more than one sense. For example, the activity in this book involving making handmade paper (see page 70) stimulates the senses with the tearing of paper, the sloshing of the water, and the feel of the wet paper.

Doing Nothing Is Actually Doing Something—Enjoying quiet time together or just sitting on a park bench can be a delightful activity for *persons* with dementia. We do not always have to be structured—life actually consists of more unstructured times. The activity Sit Beside Me (see page 180) is an excellent example of this principle.

Activities Should Tap into Physical Skills—*Persons* with dementia often retain excellent physical skills, including the ability to exercise, hike, and maintain good hand–eye coordination. Pitching and Catching (see page 111) is an example of a simple activity that keeps a *person* fit and connected to others.

Activities Are Often Initiated by Others—*Persons* with dementia typically lose the ability to initiate activities. We need to be there to help them get started. An example of this can be found in the activity Ink Paintings of Winter Trees (see page 50) in which it is important to set the activity up for the *person*, hand him or her the paint brush, and demonstrate how to begin painting.

Activities Should Be Voluntary—Most of us, including *persons* with dementia, are reluctant to do something we do not want to do. For practical and ethical reasons, a *person's* involvement in activities should be voluntary. We can gently encourage but should not be too aggressive. A good example of this concept is Let's Dance (see page 114). Dancing is a wonderful activity, and we can ask someone to dance but should respect his or her right to either participate or decline.

Intergenerational Activities Are Desirable—*Persons* with dementia can be inspired and touched by the unconditional acceptance and love of younger people. Many *persons* see young children and young adults as their own and respond to youthful exuberance. At the same time, children and young adults can be touched by the wisdom and affection shown by their elders. Sharing Life with Young Children (see page 83) gives ideas about how to create more intergenerational experiences in your activities.

Things You Think Never Will Work Often Do—We do not believe in the concept of "failure-free activities." Who leads a failure-free life? If you even could, it would mean you never took chances or tried anything new. Throughout this book, we encourage taking chances and trying new things. Encouraging *persons* with dementia to volunteer (see page 88) is a good example of this concept in practice.

Personal Care Is an Activity—Personal care is often "where the rubber meets the road" for staff and family caregivers. Are caregivers successfully getting residents dressed and bathed, or is it a constant struggle? Do staff members have time to engage in activities when they're barely keeping up with their workloads? We argue that personal care should be redefined as an activity because it adds dignity and actually helps the task get completed more quickly. Dressing and bathing (see pages 123 & 124) are examples of this new way to look at personal care.

Activities Can Be Short—Staff members often complain that they do not have enough time to do activities. We empathize with the plight of many staff whose days are consumed by personal care and other demands. Yet, Best Friends activities can be short and done throughout the day. As an example, in Chapter 1, one of the activities honors a *person's* preferred name.

Activities Are Everywhere—It is our hope that activities programs receive an adequate budget for supplies, but inspiration for activities can be found everywhere. Most of the activities in this book require minimal outlays of money to be successful. Creative staff members can also utilize everyday items and information from the library or Internet to make something out of nothing. See, for example, the creative activity around something as simple as beans (see page 37).

Activities Should also Fill Religious and Spiritual Needs—Regardless of whether a *person* with dementia has a specific faith background, everyone has spiritual needs waiting to be fulfilled. Best Friends activities celebrate a *person's* faith but also encourage staying in touch with the spirit through nature, music, and the arts. The activity Acknowledge Me (see page 5) exemplifies this with religious and spiritual components.

HOW TO USE THIS BOOK

When we began working on this book, we asked activities staff what they needed most. Almost all said that they want idea books that they can turn to and "grab and go." This book meets this need with 147 activities that can be used for 1 hour, 1 day, or even throughout a week as a "theme," for example a week's worth of activities can be planned around Summertime (see page 35).

The Best Friends Book of Alzheimer's Activities is aimed primarily at *persons* in the middle stages or course of Alzheimer's disease or related dementias. These individuals generally cannot initiate activities on their own. They need a caregiver's or staff member's help to stay connected to activities, but once they begin they can successfully participate and receive much enjoyment from their participation. As noted later in the Introduction, we also offer suggestions throughout the book for *persons* with early and late dementia.

Although much of this book is aimed at staff members working in residential or day center settings, most of the activities can easily be adapted for home settings. Friends, family, and neighbors often look for activity ideas; this book will be an inspiration for them as well as paid staff. Volunteers, in any setting, will also find the book chock full of ideas to help create a meaningful volunteer activity.

Each Activity Page

We start every activity with a brief introduction or summary in a gray, shaded box that discusses the activity in general and makes some specific remarks about how the activity particularly benefits *persons* with dementia. Read this gray box first.

The Basics

This section contains the ingredients to pull together the activity. The ingredients might include people (e.g., you and the *person* with dementia), supplies needed for an arts activity (e.g., paint, paper, tools), or a caregiving technique (e.g., find a quiet place, make eye contact). Also in this section are Variations (another activity or list of activities based on a variation of a theme discussed on the page) and Planning Tips (general tips to help activities run smoothly).

The Best Friends Way

This is where an everyday activity becomes an activity done with knack. We encourage staff members doing the activities to sample the ideas in this section so they can learn the process of converting everyday "humdrum" activities into ones with "flair." We suggest many ways to do this; you will certainly come up with more on your own!

Life Story: We start every activity with notes on this fundamental part of the Best Friends model. To deliver quality care, we need to individualize care whenever possible. In an activity setting, this can include designing activities around a *person's* past or present. It can also include acknowledging the life stories of individual members of a group, including their attitudes, values, traditions, and history.

Some of the following ingredients are also included in each activity:

The Arts: Activities are enriched when tied to the arts. This can include connecting an activity to a well-known painting, reading a poem aloud, playing classical music, or admiring a sculpture. Many of the activities also involve participating in the arts, something which can be done as actual artists or as armchair critics.

Exercise: We take note of any opportunities for stretching, walking, or other physical activities that benefit the *person* and staff member engaged in the activity. It is so valuable to keep the body moving because exercise builds strength, relieves boredom, and helps use up nervous energy.

Music: Music should be woven into as many activities as possible as it remains a source of joy for many *persons* with dementia. Even after they have lost language skills, memories of old songs are often intact. We suggest songs to sing, most of which are well known. If you don't know the lyrics, search the Internet for sites containing song lyrics or purchase songbooks.

Humor: We sometimes forget just how enjoyable laughter can be. Whether the source of humor is a joke, a humorous anecdote, or even a timely smile or gesture, laughter is a beneficial addition to almost any activity.

Early Dementia: In this section, we note whether the activity or part of the activity may be particularly helpful for *persons* with early-stage dementia. Although definitions of the stages vary, for the purposes of this book it includes individuals who have awareness of their situation and who can initiate and do activities on their own or with minimal supervision.

Late Dementia: We often forget to include *persons* with late dementia in our thinking about activities. Their ability to participate is limited but they still enjoy being in a joyful environment. Music and touch are particularly appropriate; involve them as much as possible.

Old Sayings: Experienced activities staff members know that reciting old sayings is a favorite thing to do with *persons* with dementia. Although so many memories fade, many *persons* with dementia can still complete old sayings, such as "You can lead a horse to water but . . . (you can't make it drink)." Have fun recalling old sayings and discuss their meaning.

Old Skills: Persons may recall learned motor skills or other skills they have practiced in their lives. We encourage activities that help *persons* practice these old skills, be it flipping a pancake, spinning a top, hammering a nail, or folding clothes. Successfully engaging in old skills builds a *person's* self-esteem and confidence.

Sensory: Persons with dementia benefit from activities that stimulate the five senses—touch, sound, taste, vision, and smell. Keeping this in mind can enrich many activities. For example, a simple baking activity is enhanced if the leader of the activity takes the time to encourage everyone to enjoy the smells of freshly baking bread and to do some tasting along the way.

Spirituality: Best Friends activities touch on the spiritual—whether it be acknowledging and embracing a *person's* religious faith or celebrating the *person's* spiritual nature. Spirituality often expresses itself through the arts, through music, or through long-held life values such as helping others. Although not everyone is part of a religious faith, we believe everyone has a spirit that can be touched.

Conversation: Each activity concludes with some conversation starters tied to the activity. Staff with knack don't need help in this area. Yet many staff find it helpful to see ways to talk with *persons* with dementia about the activity. We hope that these conversation starters will inspire many more questions and comments to enrich any activity.

An ounce of prevention... We assume that the staff have basic competencies and understand that supervision is important for almost all aspects of dementia care. Some activity pages note at the bottom any special precautions that need to be taken during the activity. Don't let this comment dissuade you from trying an activity; just use common sense to ensure that an activity is safe.

The Best Friends Book of Alzheimer's Activities is a rich resource of activity ideas, but it is just a starting point. Get a small group together and bring out an easel and butcher-paper pad. Pick a chapter and work through the activities together. You'll find that a group working together will easily double the number of ideas that we present on a single page. Talk about specific individuals in your program who would enjoy the activity. Make an implementation plan. Families can do similar work in home settings.

A FEW WORDS ABOUT THE INTERNET

The Internet is an endless source of information about the world we live in and a tremendous resource for staff members planning an activity. Growing numbers of activities staff have access to the Internet at work or at home. If not, most of us have public libraries we can turn to for free Internet access. The Internet allows activities professionals to:

- Find boundless information about a specific topic that can help in planning a class or writing trivia questions
- Look up lyrics to a song or words to a poem
- Discover biographical information about famous individuals (or not so famous individuals)
- Collect vintage photographs to print
- Collect music downloaded from a reputable site
- Look up a *person's* birthplace and even read his or her hometown newspaper
- Search an on-line encyclopedia
- Find old sayings and quotes
- And much more!

The Internet is also a source of continuing information about Alzheimer's disease and related disorders. "Bookmark" reputable sites such as your local Alzheimer's Association or the national Alzheimer's Association at http://www.alz.org.

We recommend updating your skills about the Internet and Internet search engines, and how they can be used for activities, but here is a basic primer. A few favorite search engines include http://www.google.com and http://www.yahoo.com. You can use these search engines to search on key words about a topic or a *person's* name. This then directs you to web sites about the topic. If you get lucky, you will immediately find the information you are looking for. If not, you may need to be even more specific in your choice of search words (e.g., if you want a recipe for wedding cake but just type in the word "weddings" you will need to sort through a lot of web sites before you ever get the recipe, if you ever do. Be more specific and type in "wedding cake recipes." Be prepared to sort out the commercial sites and extraneous sites. Patience is usually rewarded.

Sadly, there are also sites that will try to sell you questionable products or that are adult in nature or pornographic. You may consider downloading one of the software programs that screens out offensive material. Examples include programs called SurfWatch, CyberPatrol, and WebNanny.

Web sites are also a source of photographs. A good one is http://www.google.com/images. When you type a key word or name, perhaps "Frank Sinatra," you get a collection of images to sort through. Choose one, download it, and print on a color printer.

Books, both new and used, are also widely available on the web. Check your local bookstore or visit a site like http://www.amazon.com that sells millions of titles. Searches can be done by topic, which is very helpful for activities professionals.

There is also a brave new world of music downloading on the web. This is something most teenagers know more about than adults! If you are looking for an old song, there are sites that allow you to download the music (typically for a modest fee) and then play it from your hard drive and speakers or put the music into an MP3 player. One good music site is through http://www.apple.com. Click on "iTunes." Note that some materials on the web may be copyrighted. Be sure to respect copyright laws!

The web is a great adventure. Be prepared for some frustration if you have not used it before, but plunge in. To facilitate this, we have suggested key words to put into search engines throughout the book. You can use a similar approach to many of the activities found in the book.

CULTURE CHANGE

A movement is growing in the United States and around the world to consider the culture of care in our Alzheimer's programs. How do we offer quality care, stay optimistic, and be a Best Friend when reimbursements are falling, staff turnover is high, litigation is a constant worry, and regulations mount?

We propose that one way to begin to make change for the better is through activities. For *persons* with dementia, creative activities fight boredom, restore self-esteem, and reduce challenging behaviors. Successful activities help family members feel better about placement in residential care or entry into an adult day program. For staff, a new and improved, life-affirming activity program can transform a work place into a caring community, one that benefits all who live and work there.

SOME NOTES ABOUT THIS BOOK

In the book, we describe individuals with dementia with the italicized word "*person.*" We hope this reminds the reader that the *person* with dementia, despite his or her cognitive losses, is just like the rest of us, with all of our feelings and needs. This is also more economical for the reader than constantly saying "person with dementia."

We use the word *dementia* in the book to describe any person with Alzheimer's disease or a related dementia. Alzheimer's disease remains the most common cause of dementia, but we are learning more about the other dementias every day. The ideas in this book generally will work with any adult with cognitive loss, whatever his or her specific diagnosis.

We have written this book assuming that the reader has some basic knowledge about dementia and some common sense about activities. Some activities books describe the "how to's" or "basics" of the activity in such detail as to almost become laughable (e.g., pick up the song book, open the song book, find the right page in the song book, and sing). We hope we hit the right balance for the reader in being clear with our instructions, but not ridiculous.

One principle of *person*-centered care that we first wrote about in *The Best Friends Approach to Alzheimer's Care* is that every individual with dementia seems to follow his or her own unique course of illness. Some *persons* lose language skills early on; others remain surprisingly verbal. Some *persons* advance rapidly and others live with dementia for 20 years. We continue to believe that "if you've met one person with Alzheimer's disease, you've met one person with Alzheimer's disease." This suggests that it is even more important to individualize our approach to activities, give the *person* as much choice as possible, and remember that there is a *person* beneath the cloak of dementia, one who deserves our very best care.

Acknowledgments

My thanks to the staff of the Greater Kentucky/Southern Indiana Chapter of the Alzheimer's Association, especially those staff members and volunteers of the The Best Friends Center who have for more than 20 years worked daily to provide creative activities for persons with dementia. I also thank my husband, Wayne, our children, and the "grands and greats" for always being supportive.

—Virginia Bell

I appreciate the ongoing support of the Board of Directors and staff of the California Central Coast Alzheimer's Association, Santa Barbara especially Lol Sorensen, Jim Wells, and Sue Tatangelo. For their constant love and support, I thank Fred & Dorothy Troxel and Ronald Spingarn.

—David Troxel

I would like to acknowledge my family and friends for their ongoing encouragement especially Fred Cox and Jim and Judy Tincher. I also thank the Board of Directors and staff of the Greater Kentucky/Southern Indiana Chapter of the Alzheimer's Association. A special thank you to those who have given their time and creativity to developing programs in the Helping Hand Day Center: Carla Guthrie, Laurie Dorough, Laura Schneider, Jamie Kelley, Karen Dodge, Gwen Hutchinson, and Sara Marsee.

—Tonya M. Cox

I thank my family for their support and my colleagues at the Sanders-Brown Center on Aging, University of Kentucky, especially Dr. William R. Markesbery, Dr. David Wekstein, Dr. Charles D. Smith, Jeffrey N. Howe, and Jenny Cox.

—Robin Hamon

Activity Title	Page	Arts	Exercise	Nature	Evenings	Late Dementia	One-to-One	Children	For Men	Domestic	Worldly
A Clean Sweep	159		•		•					•	
Acknowledge Me	4					•	•				
A Close Shave	126						•		•	•	
Affirming Adjectives	103				•			•		•	
An Apple a Day	36			•						•	
Arranging Fresh Flowers	170			•	•	•	•			•	
Ask for My Opinion	15						•				
Baking	921				•		•	•		•	
Bathing	24						•			•	
Batting a Balloon	112		•					•			
Be Affectionate	7				•	•	•	•			
"Bean" There, Done That	37				•					•	
Bead Work	82	•	•		•		•				
Being a Volunteer	88		•	•				•	•	•	
Being in the Community	168		•	•				•	•		
Be My Valentine	85	•						•			
Bon Appetit	161				•		•			•	
Bowling	109		•	•				•			
Bright Lights, Big City	43								•		•
Brushing Teeth	129						•			•	
Camping Out	41			•							•
Caring for Pets	169		•	•	•	•	•	•	•	•	
Cars	138						•	•			•
Celebrating Cinco de Mayo	44	•				•		•		•	•
Charades	108		•					•			
Chewing the Fat	186				•		•		•		
Clay Pinch Pots	65	•						•			•
Collage	68	•			•		•				
Colors of the Rainbow	38	•					•				
Creating a Bird Sanctuary	167		•	•		•			•		
Creating One-of-a-Kind Greeting Cards	77	•					•	•		•	
Creating Wrapping Paper	80	•			•		•			•	
Dab It!	54	•	•			•	•				
Decoupage	81	•					•				
Dog Biscuits	94			•	•	•		•	•	•	
Dressing	123		•							•	
Eggshell Art	62	•		•			•				
Encourage Me	13						•				
Entertaining	93									•	•
Fabric Landscapes	60	•									
Fantasy Character Collage	59	•					•	•			
Faux Mosaics	64	•									

Activity Title	Page	Arts	Exercise	Nature	Evenings	Late Dementia	One-to-One	Children	For Men	Domestic	Worldly
Flags	146								•		•
Flashback Fashions	25									•	•
Flower Pounding	66	•	•			•	•				
Folded Paper Paintings	53	•				•	•				
Fun with Words	100						•				
Gardening	158		•	•				•	•		
Give Me a Hug	10				•	•	•	•			
Give Me Compliments	14					•	•				
Going Out to Eat	166		•				•				•
Going to Bed	131				•		•			•	
Group Exercise	115		•								
Hair Brushing & Combing	127				•	•	•			•	
Hand Care	125				•	•	•			•	
Handmade Paper	70	•	•					•	•		
Hats Off to You	39					•		•	•		•
Here Comes the Bride	29									•	
High School in the 1950's	27								•	•	
Hobbies	151				•				•	•	
Horseshoes	110		•	•			•	•	•		
Ink Paintings of Winter Trees	50	•		•			•				
Invite Me to Help	19				•	•			•		
Lace Rubbings	183	•	•		•		•			•	•
Late-Night Snack	192				•	•	•		•	•	
Laugh With Me	9				•		•	•			
Laundry	173		•		•		•		•	•	
Let Me Show You	16						•	•	•	•	
Let Me Teach You	18						•	•			•
Let's Dance	114		•				•	•		•	•
Let's Eat	121					•	•				
Listen to Me	8						•				
Listen to the Wind	26			•	•	•					•
Listening to Music	189		•		•	•	•				•
Living "Down on the Farm"	31			•				•	•	•	
Look Out the Window	17			•		•	•		•		
Lotto	106							•	•		
Make-Up	128						•			•	•
Making Bird Feeders	79		•	•					•		
Making Envelopes for Greeting Cards	78	•						•		•	
Marbling	56	•						•			
Military	142						•		•		•
Money	148						•		•	•	•
Moving and Stretching	130								•		
Music to My Ears	33	•				•	•		•		
Newspapers	149				•		•		•	•	•

Activity Title	Page	Arts	Exercise	Nature	Evenings	Late Dementia	One-to-One	Children	For Men	Domestic	Worldly
Night Owls	193		•		•		•		•	•	
Occupations	141								•		•
Old Sayings	101				•	•	•		•		
On the Road Again	30			•					•		•
Oranges with Cloves	91	•		•	•		•	•			
Painting with Bubbles	57	•						•			
Painting with Marbles	67	•					•	•	•		
Papier-Mâché Solar System	61	•		•				•	•		
Pitching and Catching	111		•	•			•	•	•		
Planning an Art Show	90	•									•
Postcard Collages	181	•		•	•		•	•			•
Potpourri	84	•		•						•	
Radio	145				•	•	•		•		•
Reading Aloud	187				•	•	•	•			
Reading Together	157				•		•	•	•		
Remember When?	182				•		•		•	•	
Remembering Childhood Games	42		•					•		•	
Reminisce With Me	12				•		•	•	•	•	•
Sandpaper Art	49	•			•		•	•			
Scrap Paper Art	58	•		•	•		•	•			
Scrap Wood Sculpture	140	•	•				•	•	•		
Sharing Life with Young Children	83		•	•		•		•			
Shopping	164		•	•			•			•	•
Sing-Along	191		•			•	•	•	•		
Sit Beside Me	180				•	•	•	•			
Sock Monkeys	86	•			•		•			•	
Sports	137		•	•					•		•
Stenciling	55	•						•			
Stop and Smell the Roses	28	•		•			•		•		
Summertime	35			•				•			
Sun Catchers	89	•		•			•	•			
Table Games	105				•		•	•	•		
Take a Walk Outside	11		•	•			•	•	•		•
Taking a Drive	163			•		•	•				
Talk about Meaningful Subjects	20				•	•	•		•		
Talking on the Telephone	165				•		•				
Tea Time	184				•					•	
Thanksgiving Blessings	40							•		•	
The Men's Club	150								•		
This is Your Life	104										
Toileting	122				•	•					
Tools of the Trade	139						•		•		•
Touring the Inside	179		•		•	•	•		•		

To staff members in long-term care
who work daily to provide creative and meaningful activities
for persons with dementia

CHAPTER ONE

Being Together
Between Structured Times

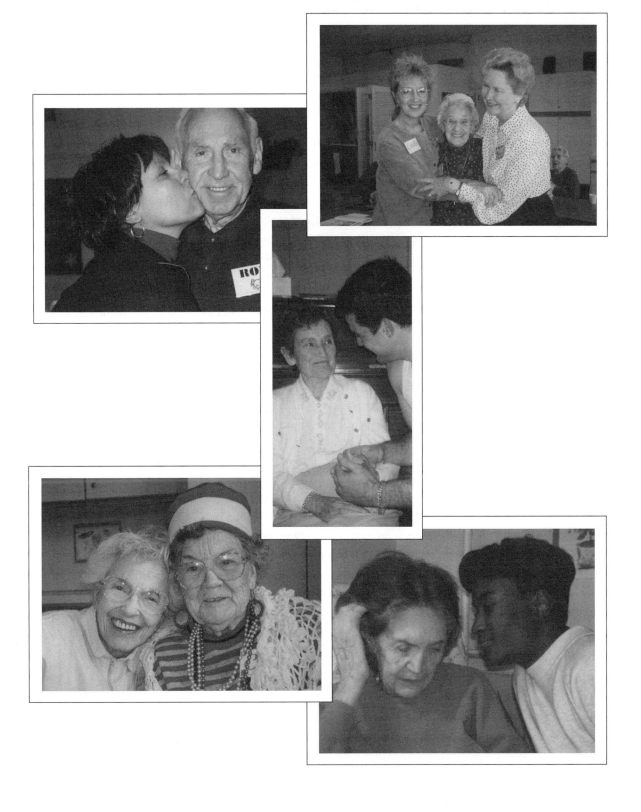

Being Together
Between Structured Times

Activity calendars set the daily agenda for most long-term care programs. These planned activities are important for many reasons, including meeting legal and licensing obligations and hopefully building a rich calendar of events for the individuals in residential or day center settings—many of whom can no longer initiate activities for themselves.

Yet for *persons* with dementia in long-term care—and for that matter, all of us—daily life is not always planned in advance and structured. Many moments occur spontaneously and activities include impromptu events or plans with just one or two friends.

For example, you might make plans to go to a play with friends months ahead of time, but your decision to have some ice cream during intermission and then to go out for coffee after the play to discuss the production may be spontaneous. In reviewing the evening, one play-goer might feel the highlight of the evening was the play, another member of the group might view the highlight as being with his or her friends, and another might have enjoyed most the post-play discussion over coffee.

As the old saying goes, "It's the little things that count," and the best programs plan their formal activities with thoughtfulness and creativity while encouraging staff to also spend time with *persons* with dementia *between* structured times. This first chapter of *The Best Friends Book of Alzheimer's Activities* is unlike any you will read in other activity books. It is designed to illuminate a new way of thinking about activities that is more in tune with everyday life. A smile, asking an opinion, and showing affection are all simple gestures, but meaningful activities for *persons* with dementia.

Many of these activities can be done in 5 minutes or fewer, or can be extended for an hour or more. These activities will help staff develop "knack" (the art of doing difficult things with ease) and to build bonds of friendship and trust. Positive relationships improve personal care routines, reduce challenging behaviors, improve dignity, and increase morale for the *person* and for staff and family members.

These activities can be done without expensive supplies and elaborate preparation. The activities are really about relationships, being with the *person* in the moment. Because these activities are not traditional, take time to work through them with staff. Creatively role-play some of the activities, and ask staff members to practice with one another. If you are a program leader, model the activities for staff with your residents, day center participants, or in home settings.

Activities in this chapter that particularly lend themselves to role playing or creative teaching include *Listen to Me*, *Give Me a Hug*, *Give Me Compliments*, and *Invite Me to Help*. Working through these activities as a group gives staff members the tools and skills to feel more relaxed with *persons* with dementia and to have more daily successes.

In this chapter, as in the rest of the book, we introduce the topic, give a few basics, encourage you to tie the activity to the *person's* life story, demonstrate the activity's benefit in a number of categories, and then bring it all together with some conversation starters. At the end of some of the activities, we offer a few words of caution under the "An ounce of prevention..." umbrella. Good luck planning to be unplanned!

CHAPTER ONE ACTIVITIES

The Basics

Even if you are busy, pause for just a few moments to acknowledge the *person* by calling him or her by name, offering a handshake or gentle touch, smiling, and making eye contact (if culturally appropriate).

Training Tip: You can model this activity at a staff meeting for all to see.

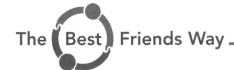

The Best Friends Way

Life Story: Use biographical information to extend the acknowledgment—for example, praise someone for his past work on a farm, for her charitable work in the community, or for being the mother of twins.

Early Dementia: Being acknowledged in a positive way can boost the morale of a *person* who is feeling the losses that accompany the diagnosis.

Late Dementia: When words become difficult to understand, a smile communicates a message without words. A *person* can often smile back, a gift to give another at a time when gift giving is limited.

Music: Greeting a *person* with a line from a familiar song, such as, "The more we get together, together, together, the more we get together, the happier are we," can be used as a ritual of acknowledgment.

Sensory: Hearing one's name and feeling a hand on the shoulder can improve a *person's* mood in a hurry.

Spirituality: Being acknowledged fulfills a spiritual need by helping a *person* reclaim his or her sense of belonging.

Conversation: Acknowledge by name, "Good morning Louise, it's great to be with you today." Tie to the life story, "Mike, it's good to see you. I remember that you were voted Teacher of the Year. Congratulations." Acknowledge with affection, "Stanley, give me one of those high fives!" While smiling, say, "Good, you are here; you add so much to my day." Begin conversation with a *person* in a wheelchair on his or her eye level, "Hello, George, that's a great-looking sweater you are wearing."

Acknowledge Me

Doesn't it feel good to be acknowledged in a special way? Because *persons* with dementia gradually lose the ability to participate in work and social activities that give them recognition, they especially appreciate acknowledgment from those around them.

An ounce of prevention...

Your efforts can backfire if the person *feels you are rushing or insincere with your acknowledgments.*

Use My Preferred Name

If you run into an old teacher at a grocery store and he or she greets you by name, how do you feel? For most of us, it's good to be recognized. In a long-term care setting, staff who use the preferred name of a *person* with dementia will usually be rewarded with smiles and good feelings.

The Basics ────────────

Ask the *person* what he or she prefers to be called. If he or she cannot respond, consult with family or friends. Teach all staff members that it only takes a few seconds to call a *person* by his or her preferred name.

Brainstorm all the ways to incorporate a *person's* preferred name into daily life, such as calling him or her by name in a greeting; introducing the *person* by name to others; discussing the origin, meaning, or correct spelling of his or her name; and addressing him or her by name before beginning personal care.

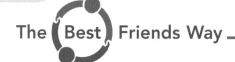

The (Best) Friends Way ────────────

Life Story: Is there a childhood nickname that the *person* recalls such as "Kitty" or "Doc?" Is the *person* named for a family member, celebrity, or friend? What is his or her middle name? Does the *person* go by initials?

Late Dementia: The recognition of one's surname (or a childhood nickname) may outlast all other memories.

Music: Songs such as "A Bicycle Built for Two" can be adapted to use other names instead of "Daisy." For example, singing "Louis, Louis, [or another name] give me your answer do. I'm half crazy all for the love of you," is a light-hearted, friendly way to use a *person's* name.

Old Sayings: "A good name is to be chosen over great riches."

Old Skills: Spelling or signing one's name is an old skill many *persons* retain long into the disease (even if his or her signature becomes wobbly). A *person* can also find joy in recognizing his or her signature on artwork, a card, or a photograph.

Spirituality: Some cultures and religious faiths have a tradition of naming children after a relative. Also, some children have names from the Bible or other religious texts. Using a preferred name honors these traditions and helps a *person* feel remembered and known.

Conversation: Ask the *person* what he or she prefers to be called, "Do you want us to call you Tom or Thomas?" The origin of a *person's* name can be talked about, "Your Dad's name was Henry. Are you named Henrietta for your father?" Reminisce, "Sadie, what did your mother call you when she needed your attention?" Use knack and give a compliment, "Happy, I know why you got your nickname! You are such a positive person."

The Basics _____

Utilize many forms of affection. Examples include hand-holding, shaking hands, a kiss on the forehead, a pat on the back, a compliment or congratulation in an affectionate way, a hug, or a gentle hand massage.

Initiate affection; hopefully the *person* will want to reciprocate. Don't overdo affection; be sincere. Until you get to know the *person*, ask for permission before initiating a physical display of affection.

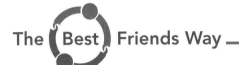 The **Best** Friends Way _____

Life Story: Is the *person* affectionate with others? Does he or she enjoy being held or hugged? Was the *person* raised in a family or culture in which affection was not openly demonstrated?

The Arts: Write poems and stories about showing love to one another.

Early Dementia: Be open to discussing the *person's* feelings around relationships and intimacy. You can also encourage attendance at an early-stage support group in which sharing of information and feelings takes place among peers.

Late Dementia: The need for affection can last throughout the disease.

Music: Sing to the *person*, "Let Me Call You Sweetheart" or "You Are My Sunshine."

Sensory: Gently rub someone's hand as you talk. Most *persons* find touch calming and reassuring.

Spirituality: Giving and receiving affection fulfills a spiritual need to love and be loved.

Conversation: Tease affectionately, "Walter, you've got the strongest handshake around—don't break my hand!" Be affectionate with words, "Marianne, thanks for being with me today on our walk. I always feel that I can talk with you about anything." Ask for support, "Mom, I really need a hug today." Reminisce about special moments of affection involving friends or family members, perhaps the first time the *person* held a baby or memories from a family reunion, birthday parties, graduations, or even a Sunday dinner.

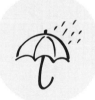

An ounce of prevention...

There can be concern about a person misjudging affection for a romantic or sexual approach. Use common sense. An isolated case should not dampen your resolve to be affectionate.

Listen to Me

Doesn't it feel good when someone really listens to you? Caregivers can fight feelings of isolation by working hard to give *persons* with dementia every chance to make themselves understood.

The Basics

Encourage staff to employ knack by practicing good listening skills. Examples include being patient, listening to words and phrases, noting the *person's* body language and facial expressions, trying to identify and understand aches and pains, and encouraging the *person* to express him- or herself.

Be sure that the environment is conducive to listening without a lot of distractions or ambient noise. Offer opportunities for staff members to practice these skills by encouraging one-to-one time sitting with *persons* in a lounge area, outdoors, or over meals.

Training Tip: Communication dos and don'ts are often successfully taught during staff role playing.

The 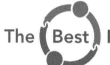 Best Friends Way

Life Story: A good listener familiar with someone's life story can sometimes "fill in the blanks" with biographical information that helps a *person* complete a thought or tell a story—for example, "Mother, your birthplace... wasn't it Kenya?"

Early Dementia: We sometimes avoid listening to *persons* who are beginning their journey of dementia by talking over them or trying to artificially cheer them up. This can inadvertently cut off conversation and be upsetting to *persons* who know their situation is more serious and who want a "listening ear."

Late Dementia: Nonverbal communication becomes most important during this time both for the *person* to communicate with staff and for the staff to communicate with the *person*.

Sensory: Seeing a concerned face can help a *person* feel comfortable expressing him- or herself verbally and nonverbally.

Conversation: Be supportive, "Take your time, Marian, I'm not in a rush. Tell me again what seems to be missing." Apologize, "I'm sorry I'm not following you. Are you looking for your brown purse?" Empathize, "I know it's frustrating right now not to be able to think of it. Let's have some hot tea while we chat." Enjoy the *person*, "That is so funny. I love that story!" Respond to the emotion behind the confused words, "I'm sorry you are sad."

An ounce of prevention...

Taking time to listen may solve a problem that is causing a person *to be angry or combative. Listening can even provide a clue about a medical problem that needs attention.*

The Basics

Collect humorous materials, such as songs, old sayings, corny jokes, pictures, stories, poems, trivia, cartoons, clothes, and objects. Embrace other forms of fun and good humor, such as clowning around, dancing a jig, give-and-take kidding, gentle teasing, and bloopers.

Use self-deprecating humor (telling a joke or story at your own expense). This can preserve dignity when embarrassing moments happen. Examples might include telling about the time you forgot to turn the oven on when preparing a Thanksgiving meal or lost your car in a parking lot.

Plan to make intentional humor a part of the day's activities. Working to create a joyful milieu elevates the mood of everyone, helps prevent challenging behaviors, and improves morale.

Laugh with Me

How many times during a day do you laugh? Laughing, and enjoying the laughter of others, is an important part of life. *Persons* with dementia often retain their sense of humor even late into the illness. They generally like to be around people who laugh a lot; laughter sends a signal that all is well.

The 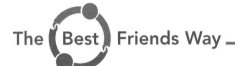 Best Friends Way

Life Story: Search the life story for humorous anecdotes. Ask a *person* to share funny stories that he or she enjoys telling. Reminisce, "Can you tell me that story about the time your pet goat ate the sofa?"

Late Dementia: Because laughter is a language without words, it is very effective in connecting to *persons* in late dementia.

Music: Sing songs that make you laugh such as "Oh Susanna" or "Whistle While You Work."

Old Sayings: "Laughter is the best medicine." "Laugh and the world laughs with you."

Sensory: Laughter not only feels good, it is physically healthy. Laughter can release pent-up emotions and calm an agitated *person*.

Conversation: Reminisce, "Norma, did you ever giggle in church when someone sang off key?" Sort through a bedroom closet, "Dad, these shoes have more holes in them than a piece of Swiss cheese!" Give a compliment, "I just love the sound of your laughter. It's so contagious." Have a friendly moment, "Do you think that joke is funny?" When you know the *person* well, don't be afraid to tease, "Harold, that is the world's corniest joke!" Use self-deprecating humor if someone comes to an activity without shoes, "I love going barefoot, too!"

An ounce of prevention...

Laugh with the person, *never at him or her.*

Give Me a Hug

Have you given someone a hug today? Most of us enjoy a good hug now and then, particularly if we are sad or upset. Many *persons* with dementia enjoy a reassuring hug to help them feel safe and secure.

The Basics

Brainstorm all the kinds and ways to give hugs:

- Gentle hugs (appropriate almost any time)
- Bear hugs (for those who are very physical)
- Side-by-side hugs (with arms around each other or just around the waist)
- Hugs from children (children give the greatest hugs)
- Two-way hugs (hugs are often initiated by the *person*)
- Group hugs (groups of friends can hug together)

The 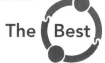 Best Friends Way

Life Story: Many *persons* come from families that had lots of physical contact or hugged each other often. Other individuals come from families or cultural traditions in which hugs were not encouraged. Try to learn the *person's* past attitude toward physical touch and hugging.

The Arts: Ask the group how they feel when hugged by a friend or someone they love. Incorporate the answers into a group poem (see Writing Poetry, page 51).

Humor: Discuss and debate whether bears really do hug!

Late Dementia: Get down to the *person's* level if he or she is in a wheelchair or in bed and give the best hug you can.

Old Saying: "I love you, a bushel and a peck, and a hug around the neck."

Sensory: The warm, soothing feel of a hug is comforting for one who feels sad, lonely, and insecure.

Conversation: Talk about the best way to be hugged, "My auntie hugged me too tight when I was a little girl. I don't like to be hugged too tight, do you?" Ask for an opinion, "Do you think men like to be hugged?" Celebrate, "Let's give each other a big hug after that long walk!" Compliment, "Georgia, you give the best hugs; keep those good hugs coming!"

An ounce of prevention...

Ask permission before beginning a hug especially if the person is new to you.

The Basics

Give thought to creating (or recommit to utilizing) outdoor space. Set it up appropriately with comfortable furniture, protection from glare, and safe surfaces for walking.

Plan for time outside just as you plan for mealtime or personal care. Use knack by inviting *persons* to join you outdoors to cut flowers, say hello to a neighborhood cat, soak up some sunshine, or watch neighborhood children play in the playground.

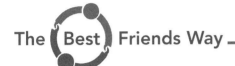

The Best Friends Way

Life Story: Did the *person* spend a lot of time outdoors, either for work, recreation, or hobbies? Did he or she walk to school or walk or hike recreationally? Did he or she enjoy window-shopping on 5th Avenue in New York or Rodeo Drive in Beverly Hills?

Exercise: Walking outside is excellent for one's general health; just a few minutes a day can add immeasurably to a *person's* mental and physical health. Don't be afraid to take a *person* outside even when the weather isn't perfect.

Late Dementia: Someone in a wheelchair can be taken outside to enjoy a beautiful day.

Music: Enjoy songs about the outdoors such as "In the Good Ole Summertime" and "Walking in a Winter Wonderland."

Sensory: Taking a walk outside is sensory rich: You can *smell* the soil after the rain and the flowers on budding trees. You can *hear* the wind whistling through the trees and the songs of the birds. You can *feel* the sun on your back and the hand holding yours. You can *see* the clouds floating by and the tall buildings. You can *taste* a muffin purchased from a neighborhood bakery.

Spirituality: Feeling connected to nature is very spiritual for many people.

Conversation: Ask for an opinion, "Eve, do you like to walk fast or slow?" or "Do you prefer warm weather or cold weather?" A discussion can be held about cars in a parking lot (e.g., license plate names, colors, "soft-top" versus "hard-top" convertibles). Seek advice, "Fred, do these look like good walking shoes?" Reminisce, "What was it like to go hiking in Yosemite?"

Take a Walk Outside

Did you ever notice how quickly a bad mood can change when you step outside on a beautiful day? For *persons* with dementia, particularly those in residential care who spend most of their time indoors, walking outside is especially valued.

An ounce of prevention...

Walking outside can be calming for a person who needs redirection from an upsetting situation.

Reminisce with Me

Most of us like to visit the past and tell old stories because reminiscing gives us time to review our lives and relive special moments. Alzheimer's disease first attacks short-term memory, so long-held memory may still be available for pleasurable reminiscence with *persons* with dementia.

The Basics

Collect as much information as possible about the *person's* life story or think about memorable times from his or her generational experiences.

Develop a list of ideas and mementos to evoke memories, such as uniforms, awards, picture books and magazines, music, recipes, and old photo albums. Encourage the *person* to reminisce with you, using meaningful moments from the life story and familiar mementos.

Variation: Develop boxes or containers on various themes such as gardening, knitting, fishing, tools, and jewelry to use for reminiscing. Pull them out when needed.

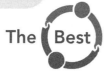

The Best Friends Way

Life Story: Knowing the *person's* life story and being creative in using it is central to reminiscing. Memories will change over time (as dementia progresses), so recall events that are meaningful to the *person* today.

The Arts: Draw pictures of early memories or make a collage from magazine pictures of some remembered experiences (examples include a collage of sights from a *person's* home town, or hobbies, or favorite foods).

Music: Use music to reminisce about where a *person* grew up, "I Left My Heart in San Francisco" or "Oklahoma." Sing a *person's* favorite song and discuss why it has special meaning to him or her.

Sensory: Aromas can trigger long-held memories.

Spirituality: Reminisce about early childhood experiences of going to church, a first communion, preparing for a bar or bat mitzvah, or other events that have given meaning and purpose to life, such as the birth of a child. Reminiscing helps keep a *person's* identity intact.

Conversation: Use the life story, "Dad, tell me about your time working in the Italian bakery." Reminisce about funny stories, "Did you really go skinny dipping?" Discuss past careers, "Was it hard work in that Pittsburgh steel factory?" Tease a woman about growing up with all boys, "Vivian, I hear that you wanted to play every sport that your brothers played!"

An ounce of prevention...

The life story can reveal topics that might be too painful to recall or, conversely, may reveal painful subjects that the person does want to talk about as part of a life review.

The Basics

Encourage the *person* during difficult times such as when the *person* is first diagnosed, is sad or lonely, needs more direction, or loses confidence.

Provide support and encouragement to help a *person* stay active and healthy—for example, to succeed in an art project, take a walk, or drink a glass of water.

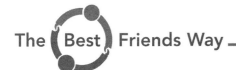

The (Best) Friends Way

Life Story: Was there a special individual or a mentor who gave encouragement to the *person* when he or she was growing up? Did the *person* serve as a role model to his or her family—for example, by encouraging his or her children to go to college?

The Arts: Encouragement helps a *person* find new artistic skills or renew old ones.

Exercise: Encouragement can be vital to help people stay physically active.

Humor: Caregivers with knack use their sense of humor often, "I can't believe that we are so good at singing those advertising jingles. If we get any better we will have to go on the road!"

Early Dementia: Sometimes *persons* at this point in the illness can encourage others with dementia by talking or writing about their experiences.

Music: Encouragement can help a *person* continue to play a musical instrument or to sing an old song. Marching music can encourage a *person* to exercise, even if he or she wants to stay seated in a chair.

Spirituality: Encourage a *person* to stay connected with his or her religious practices, "Mr. Zeff, I will read one story about Chanukah. Will you read the next story to me?"

Conversation: Encourage by saying, "You are doing so well. The cake batter just needs a few more minutes of stirring." Encouragement can lead to success in personal care, "Mr. Lopez, here is your toothbrush. I'll show you. You can brush your teeth a little longer." Encourage someone to come to a class or activity, "John, we need you at the class today. Come, let me take your arm." Encourage someone to share feelings, "Tell me more about what is upsetting you. Let's talk about it."

Encourage Me

Throughout our lives most of us were encouraged to take our first step, do well in school, seek a promotion at work, or to be kind to each other. Because of their losses, *persons* with dementia respond to a good measure of encouragement to get through their journey, or even through the day.

An ounce of prevention...

Don't fall into the trap of unrealistic expectations. If you are saying, "I know you can do it if you try harder," you may be creating a situation that will cause the person to fail and feel worse about his or her life.

Give Me Compliments

Who doesn't enjoy a compliment? A compliment can chase the blues away and help any of us feel appreciated and important. Because the self-esteem of a *person* with dementia is often diminished, a compliment is cherished even more and can focus him or her on remaining strengths.

The Basics

Brainstorm appropriate compliments for each *person*. Compliments can revolve around past achievements, clothes, or hairstyles; educational experiences; civic pride; an upbeat personality; or even well-trained pets.

Have staff members practice giving compliments to one another so that they can learn the knack of giving compliments! Encourage staff to give sincere compliments often.

Training Tip: Model giving compliments to staff members. When management points out strengths, it sets a tone that turns a workplace into a caring community.

The (Best) Friends Way

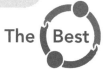

Life Story: Mine the life story for all of the ways to compliment and praise the *person*. Everyone has some accomplishment, skill, or quality worthy of a compliment.

Humor: A compliment can be humorous, "You are the best thing since sliced bread."

Late Dementia: A *person* responds to the tone of a caregiver's voice or his or her facial expression.

Old Skills: *Persons* can give compliments and get much pleasure in doing so.

Sensory: Compliments can be given while stroking a *person's* hair or gently massaging his or her hand.

Conversation: Reassure, "You're doing just fine. I'm proud of your determination." Build self-esteem, "Ray, you and your Rotary Club helped so many children around the world." Remind a *person* of his or her special expertise, "You are a great stone mason; your patios and walkways have made our town so beautiful." A compliment can encourage, "Just one more step and you will be there. I knew you could make it to your chair." A compliment can build self-esteem, "Linda, you are wearing a beautiful hat today. I love it! It makes you look so sophisticated."

An ounce of prevention...

Use a compliment to change the mood or to "disarm" someone who is agitated or upset. It can change a person's mood very quickly . . . Note however, compliments should not be overdone, childish, or otherwise inappropriate.

The Basics

Ask *persons* for their opinions on the events of the day, including menus and clothing choices and things such as the latest hair styles of the staff or whether it is going to rain.

Asking an opinion shows respect. If we make all of the decisions for a *person*, then he or she can become frustrated and angry.

Training Tip: Brainstorm topics to ask *persons* their opinions about.

Ask for My Opinion

Have you ever participated in a public opinion poll? When someone asks us our opinion it gives importance to our lives; someone cares about what we think. *Persons* with dementia can feel this same sense of importance and pride when someone asks their opinion.

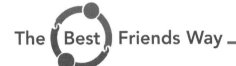

The Best Friends Way

Life Story: Ask a cook about a recipe, ask a sports fan about a favorite team, or ask a golfer to offer his or her opinion of your golf swing.

The Arts: Go to a street fair or a museum and ask the *person* his or her opinion about the artwork. Listen to music and be armchair critics.

Humor: In a humorous tone say, "I always have an opinion on everything."

Early Dementia: *Persons* with early dementia need to have as much self-determination as possible. It is important to ask their opinions often.

Late Dementia: Don't assume *persons* with late dementia cannot give an opinion. Watch for nonverbal cues signaling their opinions about their favorite foods or how they prefer to be bathed.

Sensory: Ask an opinion about the taste of dinner or the scent of a new hand cream.

Conversation: Talk about your wardrobe, "Molly, do you like this dress on me?" or "Does this tie match my shirt?" Use open-ended questions, "What would you suggest?" or "What do you think?" Ask about a purchase in a seed catalog, "Do you think tulips would be nice in our garden?" Ask an opinion about a young couple, "Yulan, how long should two people know each other before they marry?"

An ounce of prevention...

Avoid overly controversial topics. When you ask for an opinion, be prepared for the sometimes all-too-candid response; persons might tell you they don't like your new outfit or hairdo!

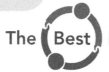

Let Me Show You

How often do you show off your hobbies, collectibles, or other prized possessions? It feels good when someone takes an interest in your world. Asking a *person* with dementia to show you his or her special things can be very pleasurable and a source of pride.

The Basics

For caregiving in a *person's* home, become familiar with each of his or her favorite possession(s). Invite the *person* to show a specific possession, "I understand you painted watercolors. May I see your collection?"

For *persons* in residential care, identify something special that they have brought into the facility from their homes. Alternatively, ask to see a recently created art project that he or she may have proudly hung.

The Best Friends Way

Life Story: Favorite possessions vary from *person* to *person* but may include: family photos; an afghan; a hand-painted picture; awards, badges, or certificates of appreciation; a rock collection; a new purse; a musical instrument; a favorite chair; or a family Bible.

Late Dementia: A *person* may be able to show you his or her unusual watch or the fabric of his or her hand-made sweater.

Music: Listen to or sing, "(These Are a Few of) My Favorite Things" from the movie *The Sound of Music*.

Sensory: Handling a beautiful ring or bracelet is an opportunity to touch and massage a hand.

Spirituality: Ask the *person* to show you his or her Bible, menorah, prayer beads, or other religious items.

Conversation: This is a perfect time to reminisce, "Mark, where did you get that old fiddle?" or "Tell me about this photograph." Build self-esteem, "Sharon, I'd love to see a copy of the book you wrote. I understand it was a bestseller!" Kidding and teasing with *persons* about some of their things can be fun, "That ceramic elephant is so old that it must have been on Noah's ark." Give praise, "Look at these tiny stitches. Ginny, you really know how to quilt!"

An ounce of prevention...

Not everyone will want to show off their possessions, in part because persons with dementia can become fearful that their things will be taken by others. Use common sense and your best judgment in this arena.

The Basics

One element of caregiving knack is learning the ability to make something out of nothing. Here we make the most from a view out a window: birds perched on a limb; blue sky and white puffy clouds; children playing; a gardener at work; squirrels on the telephone line and the pet rabbit nibbling the grass; sunshine, shadows, snow, and maybe a snowman; spring flowers, rain, and a rainbow; an oak tree filled with acorns and a beautiful sunset; people passing by; and tall buildings.

Make sure you have some comfortable chairs next to the window, because the *persons* may want to enjoy the view by themselves.

Look Out the Window

How many times have you paused and enjoyed a view out of a window? This can make for a relaxing moment or provide endless free entertainment! Looking out a window with a friend who provides commentary can be enriching and provide much to talk about for *persons* with dementia.

The 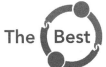 Best Friends Way

Life Story: Relate things seen out the window to a *person's* life story. Seeing a hot dog stand or tall building can remind someone of the city where he or she grew up. Changes in weather or seasons can be good starting points for reminiscing about where a *person* has previously lived.

The Arts: Write a poem or make up a story about what you see outside the window. Paint a picture or compose a simple drawing from the scene.

Exercise: Take time to clean the windows together, using an appropriate spray, paper towels, cloths, or even a squeegee.

Humor: Laugh about the squirrels playing tag or other humorous things you observe.

Old Skills: Counting cars or people passing by rehearses an old skill.

Sensory: Feeling the warmth or cold of the glass can awaken the sense of touch.

Conversation: Initiate spotting a bird, "Look at that beautiful red cardinal." Ask an opinion, "Do you like to walk in the rain?" Debate, "Mr. Douglas, what's the fastest way to get around in this city? By bus or by car?" Talk about the season of the year, "You can tell it is spring time. Look how green the grass is now." Laugh together, "Is that a snow man or a snow woman?"

Let Me Teach You

Are you a teacher? You may not be a teacher in the sense of developing a formal curriculum or teaching an hour-long class, but you have the potential to share with others a unique skill or talent. Many *persons* with dementia seem to transcend their disability when teaching others a familiar skill or art.

The Basics

Initiate the activity by inviting the *person* to teach his or her particular skill. Examples might include how to spin a wooden top; tie a knot that won't slip; polish stones; make a quilt; crochet and knit; make blackberry jam; cook chicken and dumplings; can dill pickles; play a mouth harp; dance a jig; whistle; build a moonshine still; count to 10 in various languages (even sign language); make a corncob pipe; recite poems, nursery rhymes, old sayings, and truisms; or describe the uses of medicinal herbs.

You may need to help set up the teaching experience and encourage the *person* along the way. Many of the previous examples are learned skills that may survive dementia longer than teaching more intellectual material such as history or literature.

The 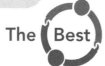 Best Friends Way

Life Story: Be a detective. Look at the life story for clues to interests and ideas that a *person* still has intact and would enjoy teaching another.

Exercise: A *person* who is a retired coach can teach a volunteer how to throw a football. A golfer can help others practice their swing. All of these activities involve stretch, movement, and exercise!

Early Dementia: Teaching a particular hobby or skill is particularly fulfilling for *persons* with early dementia.

Old Skill: Teaching is an old skill and is well rehearsed through the years.

Spirituality: To be respected as a teacher gives purpose and meaning to one's life. It leaves a legacy for future generations.

Conversation: Ask for help, "Edna Carroll, I can never tie my scarf properly. Can you teach me how?" or "Show me that dance step one more time?" Encourage the sharing of hobbies, "Paul, would you bring your beautiful polished stones for us to see? We would like for you to tell us how you polish them." Provide a cue that evokes an old skill, "Sophie, can you tell us how to count to 10 in Polish again?"

An ounce of prevention...

Be prepared to step in and help out if a person loses his or her train of thought while teaching or showing others.

18

The Basics ───────────────

Make an inventory of all the ways *persons* may be able to help. Brainstorm examples such as: setting up or moving chairs, handing out napkins, serving tea or coffee, tasting or seasoning the soup, helping make a bed, watering plants, feeding fish, and gardening. Include *persons* in as much of the everyday routine as possible.

Invite Me to Help

It feels good when we are invited to help a friend, family member, or colleague. *Persons* with dementia are left with fewer and fewer ways to contribute; caregivers with knack empathize and plan ways to invite the *person* to help.

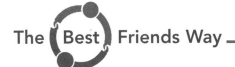

The (Best) Friends Way ───────────────

Life Story: What in the *person's* life story would suggest that you invite him or her to help you with a certain thing? Maybe they have been farmers or gardeners, cooks, builders, homemakers, artists, accountants, nurses, or teachers or have engaged in many other careers and would love to be invited to share their expertise to help out. Consider another possibility; some individuals may not have a tradition or pattern of helping others or may feel that they are "retired" and don't want to work.

Exercise: Pushing a cart, accompanying staff on a mission, and working in a garden are all ways to incorporate exercise into a helping encounter.

Early Dementia: Some *persons* may be working at paying jobs early in the illness. If this becomes impossible, they may still want to try volunteer activities including serving meals to the homeless or helping a nonprofit organization with office work.

Old Skills: Asking a *person* to help evokes old social graces and might encourage him or her to do something he or she otherwise would not attempt.

Spirituality: An invitation to help can make a *person* feel valued as a contributing member of society.

Conversation: Be generous with compliments, "Thanks for holding those towels for me. I needed your helping hands." Reminisce while getting the room ready for worship, "José, I remember that you volunteered as an usher. Would you help me pass out the programs today?" Ask for help, "Maria, would you help me water the plants. They're looking a little dry." Encourage a *person* to join a group activity, "Would you turn the pages of the sheet music for me while I play this song?"

An ounce of prevention...

When asking for help, choose wisely to try to match the request with the person's *ability to help.*

Talk About Meaningful Subjects

Do you have someone in your life who is a confidant? Having a trusted friend to confide in can help you cope with many of life's challenges. Many *persons*, especially those with early dementia, have a need to talk to someone about meaningful subjects.

The Basics

Persons may want to talk about meaningful subjects such as their travels, career, family, and their challenges with Alzheimer's disease.

Persons may also enjoy debating broad philosophical topics or truisms. Some examples include Can you judge a book by its cover? Is it better to give than receive? Are men different than women? Is a dog really man's (and woman's) best friend? Do children grow up faster today than they used to?

The 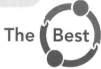 Best Friends Way

Life Story: Getting to know each *person's* life story gives clues for topics of conversation that are most satisfying.

The Arts: Going to a poetry or book reading, a modern dance performance, or a ballet is an adult activity that respects a *person's* past interests.

Early Dementia: *Persons* with early dementia often complain that the conversation is too shallow. They want to address meatier subjects and talk about their illness. They may want to discuss how memory loss is affecting their daily lives, worries about their caregivers, and what they see ahead of them.

Spirituality: To have a friend who listens and converses with you about meaningful things fulfills a spiritual need to be understood.

Conversation: Empathize, "It must be very difficult to have to give up driving. I can understand why you are sad at times." Celebrate, "I'm glad that you told me about your wonderful daughter. You must enjoy seeing her more now that you live closer to her." Enjoy travel talk, "Let's continue that conversation about your trip to Pompeii. I like archeology too, and I love hearing all about your visit to the ancient ruins." Validate feelings, "I know you are worried about your husband and all the work he's doing for you nowadays. Tell me more about your husband Kenneth."

An ounce of prevention...

If the person has a concern or unresolved life issue that is beyond your ability to help, seek appropriate guidance from a mental health professional.

CHAPTER TWO

Recreating the Classroom Experience

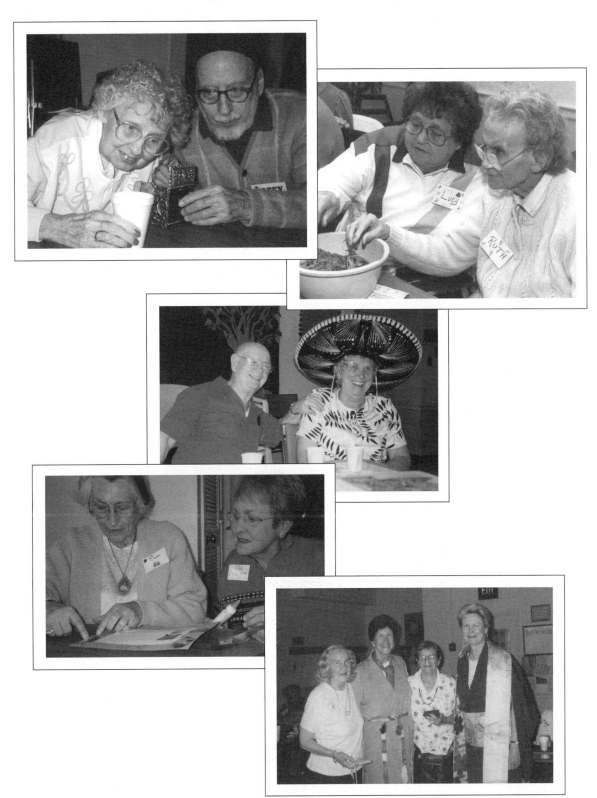

Recreating the Classroom Experience

Every day presents opportunities to learn something new. From the time we wake up until the time we go to bed, we might learn a new word; information or trivia from a book, current news from a report, web site, or e-mail; a different route to drive home; or something new about one of our friends. Being in a classroom setting evokes these traditions of learning. This chapter helps you plan classes focusing on sensory-rich, interesting topics for *persons* with dementia to explore. The classes are built around information and trivia about specific subjects that are combined with items and props to stimulate discussion.

Persons with Alzheimer's disease or a related dementia typically cannot retain the new information discussed in class, yet caregivers with knack understand why this activity is so valuable. Even if *persons* do not retain the information discussed in class, they still enjoy the *experience* of learning. They also enjoy the sense of community and success that comes from a class setting, and these happy feelings, "emotional memories," can last long after the class is over.

When you teach the class, begin with some information about the topic or use trivia (fun, short facts) that can be revealed or formed into questions. For example, in the activity entitled *Summertime*, you can describe the length of the season and time of year, talk about how the seasons are reversed in different hemispheres, and then present trivia. Here are some trivia questions you can ask: When was the bikini introduced? (1946); Where is the hottest place in the USA? (Death Valley); What popular summer drink uses bourbon? (mint julep). Props might include everything from vintage bathing suits to beach balls to cold slices of watermelon.

To promote successful classroom activities, consider the following:

- Ideally these activities will be done in small groups, yet we have seen larger groups succeed with additional staff and volunteer support.
- The right questions make better discussion and involvement. Create questions that involve genuinely interesting facts and ones that will get a good-natured debate or conversation going.
- Incorporate each *person's* life story into the topic as much as possible.
- Stimulate all of the senses. Don't limit the classroom session to talking and reminiscing about a certain subject. Bring in items that involve taste, touch, smell, hearing, and rich visuals.
- Don't make the session too lengthy. Plan to spend only 30–45 minutes on each topic. Even if you find lots of information or items to share, you need not use everything in one session.
- Be flexible! If you plan a topic and the group starts to talk about something else or heads in another direction, just go with them! You can always do the planned topic at another time.
- Be prepared! Even a short amount of time researching topics in the library, at a book store, or on the Internet will make everything go better.

- Model ahead of time these classroom activities for staff. It will be fun, staff will learn more about one another, and it will encourage everyone to think about the importance of creative activities.
- Consider creating a "class topic" committee to research and write future topics. Family members or community volunteers are ideal choices for such a committee.
- Try "theme weeks." You can take almost any topic in this chapter and have fun with it over a week. Parcel out a few different trivia questions every day, spend the week creating a themed bulletin board, or utilize some of the material suggested in each of this chapter's activities over the course of a week.

As you conduct the activities in this chapter, look around the room. You will see expressions of surprise, smiles, laughter, and nods of recognition not only from *persons* but also from staff members and family members who are present. These topics have genuine interest for most everybody—many *persons* with long-term memory will share rich insights into the past. Many staff members from differing cultures and hometowns can add their own comments, hobbies, traditions, and stories to the mix. Family members may be inspired to suggest future topics for discussion. In fact, when you think of the world of potential classroom topics, it would be possible to offer a different class every week and every day.

CHAPTER TWO ACTIVITIES

The Basics

Before Class: Collect information and trivia about fashions. Helpful Internet keywords include: fashion, vintage fashion, zoot suit, antique costumes, bell-bottom jeans, pill-box hat. Obtain vintage clothing from consignment shops, garage sales, or a volunteer's closet and books on fashion (preferably with lots of pictures, e.g., flapper costumes from the 1920s).

At Class Time: Have group participants and staff model the fashions or pass around picture books and photographs. Share fun fashion facts, or ask the group to answer prepared trivia questions regarding fashion, such as "What is a zoot suit?" Discuss and reminisce about the old fashions.

The 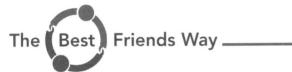 Friends Way

Life Story: Find out if any participants in the class once worked in retail or were tailors or seamstresses. Did any members of the group have a particular wardrobe or uniform required for their job?

Humor: Joke about fashion mishaps such as the time that someone appeared at a formal dinner wearing two different-colored shoes. Tease someone about owning 200 pairs of shoes.

Music: Use songs related to clothing and fashion such as "Alice Blue Gown"; "Easter Bonnet"; or "Five Foot Two."

Old Sayings: Caregivers with knack understand that old sayings are often part of a *person's* long-term memory. It gives a *person* pleasure to recall and discuss the meaning of old sayings like: "A stitch in time saves nine," "dressed to the nines," or "clotheshorse."

Sensory: Feel textures such as silk and burlap, and look at colors and patterns.

Spirituality: Discuss the meaning of the saying, "He would give you the clothes off of his back."

Conversation: Ask an opinion, "Do you like that style?" Ask for help, ""How do you sew on a button?" Have a friendly debate, "Do the clothes make the man?" Laugh together, "Can you believe that we thought those bell-bottom pants looked so great? I can't believe we wore those!" Reminisce, "Elizabeth, I know you lived in London during the 1960s. Did you ever meet that famous fashion model, Twiggy?"

Flashback Fashions

Looking at fashions of long ago helps us remember certain times or events in our lives. *Persons* with dementia can discuss fashions, model fashions for the group, or simply enjoy the show.

An ounce of prevention...

Sometimes persons *will mistakenly claim items of clothing as their own. If this happens, gently redirect or be patient and take the items back quietly at a later time.*

25

Listen to the Wind

This class celebrates something that is almost always present, but something we do not pay enough attention to—the wind. During the class, there are lots of opportunities for feeling the wind, hearing music inspired by wind, or listening to each other whistle. This session is sensory rich for *persons* with dementia.

The Basics

Before Class: Collect information and trivia about the wind. Internet keywords include: wind instruments, windmills, wind chimes, weather.

Also collect items related to the wind, including wind chimes made of various materials, whistles, empty glass bottles, and windsocks. Gather together some musical instruments that use wind such as a clarinet, flute, or recorder and other wind-related items, such as kites, pictures of windmills, or amateur weather stations/weather vanes.

At Class Time: Listen to the wind chimes. Look at the windsocks. Use a fan to demonstrate how they work. Play the wind instruments. Try making music by blowing across the opening of a bottle. Have everyone in the group try to whistle. Discuss information and trivia related to the wind.

The 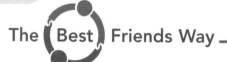 Best Friends Way

Life Story: Tie a class discussion to your knowledge of those members of your group who play a musical instrument. If any members of your group were pilots, have them share their flying experience and how the wind affects flight. Did anyone ever see a windmill in Holland?

The Arts: Enjoy a live concert or recording of classical music involving wind instruments.

Exercise: On a pretty day, try flying a kite together.

Humor: Laugh with each other as you try to whistle or blow across the opening of a bottle.

Old Sayings: "Gone with the wind." "Wind in the willows."

Sensory: Listen to the sounds made by musical instruments and wind chimes. Explore the different materials of the wind chimes.

Spirituality: In the Native American tradition, natural elements, such as the wind, have a sacred meaning. Ask participants to share their spiritual or religious beliefs about natural elements.

Conversation: Speculate, "How do you know which way the wind is blowing?" Take a survey, "What do you think of the wind chimes? Which one sounds best?" Joke, "Do you believe those weather forecasters can really predict the weather?" Share some trivia, "Some people believe that when a butterfly flaps its wings it creates the weather around the world. Could that be true?" Reminisce, "Miss Laura, was it your chore to hang the clothes out to dry?"

The Basics _____

Before Class: Collect information and trivia about schools and the 1950s. Internet keywords include: school days, 1950s fashion, music from the 1950s. Check web sites of schools that your group attended.

Also collect items related to school, including: 1950s-style lunch boxes, rulers, old school books, school supplies, letterman's jacket, a Hula-Hoop, yearbooks, old class photos, chalk board, or a jump rope or basketball to reminisce about sports and gym class.

At Class Time: As the group leader, dress in 1950s attire (poodle skirt and bobby socks or jeans and leather jacket). Pass around the items you've collected. Lead the group in discussion and reminiscence. Use a chalkboard during part of the activity to evoke the classroom experience; encourage everyone to hold the chalk and write on the board. Use different colors of chalk.

Variations: If several members of your group are from the same school, focus a class discussion about that particular school. Also, you can adapt this activity to different decades.

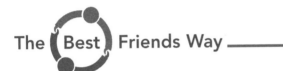 The **Best** Friends Way _____

Life Story: Learn about the *person's* school experiences. Did anyone wear a school uniform? Did anyone attend school in the 1950s? Does someone remember being taught by Catholic nuns? Did anyone have a favorite teacher? Note if any members of the group were teachers. Did any group member win special student awards or scholarships? Highlight those achievements. Did anyone play basketball for his or her school?

Exercise: Enjoy chair exercises to the tunes of music popular in the 1950s.

Humor: Discuss playing hooky. Does anyone want to admit he or she did it?

Music: Listen to music from the 1950s and reminisce about high school dances.

Old Sayings: "An apple for the teacher." "The three Rs at school—reading, 'riting, and 'rithmetic."

Sensory: Smell sticks of chalk. Feel the spiral and paper of a notebook. Touch a basketball and listen to it bounce.

Conversation: Explore a memory, "Did you have a large graduating class from high school?" Ponder, "Would you like to be back in school again?" Connect to the life story, "Lucy, when you taught school did you have a favorite student?" Reminisce, "Professor Newton, did you ride the subway to your school in the Bronx?"

High School in the 1950s

Almost everyone has had some kind of school experience. Because this was such a rich, developmental time for all of us, *persons* with dementia often enjoy talking about school days.

An ounce of prevention...

Be sensitive to those members in your group who may have had a bad experience with school or failed to graduate due to life circumstances.

Stop and Smell the Roses

Flowers add joy and beauty to our lives. *Persons* with dementia may find discussing and working with beautiful flowers particularly enjoyable and rewarding.

The Basics

Before Class: Collect information and trivia about flowers. Internet keywords include: gardening, wildflowers, flowers, *Farmer's Almanac*, roses.

Also collect books on flowers (preferably those with lots of pictures) or a *Farmer's Almanac*; fresh flowers; scissors; vases; and gardening tools such as gloves, hats, rakes, or spades.

At Class Time: Pass around the flowers. Ask the names of them. Talk about the varieties of flowers and how they can be named for famous people (e.g., Queen Elizabeth or Mr. Lincoln rose). Share other fun facts or create trivia questions based on your Internet or library research. Play a Flower Lotto Game (see page 108). Create a flower arrangement or arrangements (see Arranging Fresh Flowers on page 170).

Variation: Focus on a specific flower each day of the week.

The 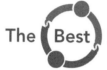 Best Friends Way

Life Story: Find out if the *person* gardens as a hobby. What flowers has the *person* grown in his or her garden? What is the *person's* favorite flower? Is someone named for a flower?

The Arts: Use fresh flowers for "flower pounding" activity (see page 66). Create a crossword puzzle or other word game from names of flowers.

Exercise: Take a walk to enjoy springtime wildflowers.

Humor: "I don't have a green thumb, I can't keep anything growing!"

Music: Sing, "When You Wore a Tulip" or "April Showers."

Old Sayings: "Mary, Mary quite contrary, how does your garden grow?" "Roses are red, violets are blue. . . "

Sensory: Smell the flowers and feel their petals, stem, and leaves.

Conversation: Discuss, "What types of flowers are traditionally used for Easter, Valentine's Day, or weddings?" Ask an opinion, "Joe, how do you keep bugs from eating your roses?" Research together, "Let's see what the *Farmer's Almanac* tells us about planting flowers." Explore a topic, "Lydia, I wonder how they use flowers to make perfume."

An ounce of prevention...

Avoid toxic plants and be watchful about potential allergies.

The Basics

Before Class: Collect information and trivia about weddings. Internet keywords include: weddings, wedding customs, wedding traditions.

Also collect items related to weddings: a dress, tuxedo, wedding bells, photos, wedding music, flowers, cake toppers, bridal magazines, and wedding cakes.

At Class Time: Encourage participants to look at the photos and bridal magazines. Pass around the items and talk about each one. Model a wedding dress. Serve a slice of wedding cake and play some wedding music. Ask trivia questions or present fun facts about weddings.

Variations: Discuss wedding traditions and customs from different cultures and countries. Sometimes a day center or residential care program will have a staff (or family) member who is getting married and willing to share his or her experience with the group. Perhaps they will even renew their vows in the program so that everyone can "attend the wedding."

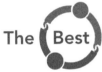

The Best Friends Way

Life Story: Learn about the wedding experiences and traditions of *persons* in the group. Some people may have had a civil ceremony that was small; others may have had a large church wedding. Did anyone elope? Did anyone have a particular song at his or her wedding? Where did a couple go on their honeymoon?

Humor: Laugh about wedding day mishaps such as the cake toppling over.

Music: Listen to such favorites as "For Me and My Gal," "I Want a Girl," and "Get Me to the Church on Time" as well as traditional wedding music such as "The Wedding March."

Old Sayings: "Something old, something new, something borrowed, something blue."

Sensory: Enjoy the feel of the fabric of the wedding dress. Taste wedding cake. Smell the flowers. Listen to the wedding music and ringing of the bells.

Spirituality: Ask participants and their caregivers to share their own cultural and religious traditions around weddings with the group.

Conversation: Discuss wedding superstitions such as throwing the bouquet, not seeing the bride before the ceremony, or throwing rice. Ask for information, "Mrs. White, what is a bride's hope chest?" Ask for advice, "Margie, what is the recipe for a good marriage?" Ask people to share ideas for a toast to the bride and groom. Discuss famous couples: Adam & Eve, Prince Philip & Queen Elizabeth, George Burns & Gracie Allen, Humphrey Bogart & Lauren Bacall, Elizabeth Taylor & Richard Burton.

Here Comes the Bride

Most people have had experience with weddings, whether their own or that of a family member or friend. Weddings are one of life's milestones and an important ritual for many *persons* with dementia.

An ounce of prevention...

Be cautious in this class because some people may have sad memories regarding marriage.

On the Road Again

Vacations hold special memories whether we took them as children with our parents or later in life. Because vacations are often full of unusual and sometimes even dramatic experiences, *persons* with dementia may recall some aspects of their vacations.

The Basics

Before Class: Collect information and trivia about vacations and travel. Internet keywords include: travel, vacation, or a specific city such as Miami or Honolulu.

Also collect old postcards from different places, travel brochures, maps, globes, or some vacation items: camera, book, clothes, passport, and sunglasses. Provide a flip chart and markers.

At Class Time: Pass around photos and postcards of vacation destinations. Reminisce about past vacations. Play a game of places to visit, asking questions such as "Where am I if I am going to a luau?" or "Where am I if I am looking out from the top of the Empire State Building?" List on a flip chart places that class participants have been for a vacation. Talk about places they would like to visit. Share other fun facts or trivia about travel.

Variation: Take a fantasy trip across the United States displaying road maps, discussing various cities, regional attractions, local foods, and more along the way.

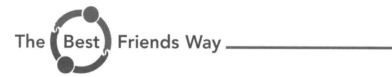

The (Best) Friends Way

Life Story: Learn about favorite vacation spots or travel destinations of the members of your group. Who in your group has been a big traveler? Do members of your group have interesting childhood vacation memories?

The Arts: Make a collage using postcards (see page ??) Read Robert Frost's poem, "The Road Less Traveled."

Humor: Talk about funny mishaps, "When I got off the airplane, I discovered I had been booked to Portland, Maine and not Portland, Oregon!"

Music: Sing songs about different places such as: "Carolina in the Morning," "Deep in the Heart of Texas," "California Here I Come," or "My Old Kentucky Home."

Sensory: Looking at pictures and postcards from vacation can remind *persons* of the sights and sounds of faraway places.

Conversation: Discover memories from the past, "Clyde, how did you travel to vacation spots: by car or by plane?" or "What was it like to fly across the country in the 1950s?" Ask for advice, "What are the essentials to pack when going on vacation?" Debate, "Is it better to relax during a vacation or see as much as you can?" Dream, "Jenny, if you could take a vacation anywhere, where would you go?"

The Basics

Before Class: Collect information and trivia about farming and agriculture. Internet keywords include: farm life, farmhouse, milking cows.

Also collect items related to farming: an old milk bucket, a butter churn, an egg basket, farm tools, pictures of farm life, a *Farmer's Almanac*, and fresh vegetables.

At Class Time: Pass around the items and talk about each one. Offer trivia questions. Discuss life experiences related to farming. Read passages from the *Farmer's Almanac* and debate and discuss. Taste fresh vegetables such as a tomato or cucumber.

Variations: Celebrate intergenerational activities by inviting the Future Farmers of America to come and visit the class to discuss their program and activities.

Living "Down on the Farm"

Farm life was a way of living for many people. This class discussion allows *persons* with dementia who grew up on farms or lived in rural settings to share their experiences. For the rest of us, it's an opportunity to experience a slice of life that is slowly disappearing from many countries.

The 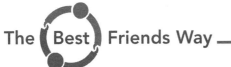 Best Friends Way

Life Story: Review life stories to see which *persons* lived on farms. Who had a favorite relative who lived on a farm? What chores was a *person* responsible for?

The Arts: Create a farm-themed word game.

Humor: Joke about using an outhouse or the silly things farm animals can do.

Music: Listen to recordings of "Shine On Harvest Moon" or "Green Acres."

Old Sayings: "Planting by the light of the moon." "You reap what you sow."

Sensory: Look at an old milk bucket. Feel the cold metal, knock on the bucket to hear its sound. Feel the texture of the egg basket. Enjoy the smell, taste, and feel of fresh vegetables.

Spirituality: Discuss the cycles of growth and harvest, which are symbolic of life. Talk about how being productive and sharing your produce with others is spiritually rewarding.

Conversation: Reminisce, "What time did you wake up on the farm? Did a rooster crow to wake you up? What crops did you grow?" While looking at the farm tools ask, "Paul, what do you do with this tool?" Recall together, "When does the harvest moon take place? Did you ever milk a cow, gather eggs, or feed the pigs? How do you milk a cow? How many eggs does a chicken lay each week? Did you follow the *Farmer's Almanac*? What types of information and advice does it provide?"

Trip to the Ocean

The ocean can be a very serene and tranquil setting. Many of us have memories from visiting the beach. This topic provides an opportunity for *persons* with dementia to relive the sensory experiences of nature through feeling the sand, listening to the sounds of the ocean, and looking at beautiful pictures of beaches.

The Basics

Before Class: Collect information and trivia about the ocean. Internet keywords include: tide charts, oceans, surfing, best beaches.

Collect items such as: a globe of the earth, an atlas showing the various oceans, a book featuring ocean photography, or items related to the beach: conch shell, beach ball, sand bucket and shovel, pictures of the ocean and beach, sand dollar, surf board, and sand in a bottle.

At Class Time: Begin the class by looking at the globe or atlas and identifying the major oceans of the world. Pass around the beach items and discuss each one. Enjoy the colors and textures. Try to hear the ocean in the seashell. Use information to discuss trivia questions related to the ocean such as the difference between a dolphin and a porpoise. Discuss ocean experiences such as sailing, walking on the beach, and going on a cruise.

The 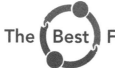 Best Friends Way

Life Story: Was anyone a sailor, or did anyone work in a shipyard? Did anyone scuba dive, snorkel, or surf? Did anyone travel to the beach? Did a *person* grow up on the east coast and call the oceanfront "the shore" or west coast and talk about "the beach?" Celebrate the diversity of your center by discovering which ocean people were born closest to. See who enjoyed taking cruises.

The Arts: Create a fabric seascape (see page 60). Have an outrageous beach costume day at the program and encourage the wearing of loud Hawaiian shirts or muumuus.

Music: Play music with the sound of waves crashing in the background (as on relaxation tapes/CDs) or sing "Red Sails in the Sunset" and "My Bonnie."

Sensory: Look at seashells. Listen to the ocean in a conch shell. Bring in beach sand for individuals to run through their fingers or step into barefoot.

Spirituality: Use a poem or descriptive painting to lead a discussion about the majesty of the ocean.

Conversation: Reminisce, "Taylor, did you ever swim in the ocean? Walk on the beach? Did you ever go deep-sea fishing? Have you ever collected seashells? What types of shells did you find?" Discuss some trivia, "Maura, I wonder how sand is made? What makes the different colors?" Other questions could include, "How many oceans are there? Can we name them? (Indian, Pacific, Atlantic, Arctic) Which ones have you visited?"

The Basics _____

Before Class: Collect information and trivia on musical instruments. Internet keywords include: musical instruments (by type), symphony, philharmonic.

Also collect musical instruments, particularly ones that are easy to bring to class (e.g., harmonica, recorder, tambourine, castanets, guitar, autoharp, bells, bongo drums).

Persons might also enjoy photographs of famous musicians with their instruments (available on old album covers or from Internet sites).

At Class Time: Look at the photographs of musicians and discuss. Pass the instruments around. Play the instruments. Allow each *person* to play at least one instrument. Talk about the sounds that each makes. If possible, have a musician come in and give a short (15–20 minutes) concert. Mix it up. Invite a choir, folk singer, or even a rock-and-roll band in for a concert (if they aren't too outrageous!).

Music to My Ears

Many people have had the opportunity to learn to play a musical instrument or appreciate listening to music. This session uses musical instruments to create a rich activity for *persons* with dementia, whose musical appreciation often remains strong throughout their illness.

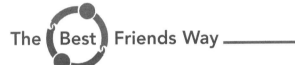

The (Best) Friends Way _____

Life Story: Is the *person* from a musical family? Find out each *person's* favorite type of music and whether he or she took music lessons. Did he or she ever play in a school band? Research folk instruments that relate to a *person's* cultural background (a zither from Eastern Europe, a sitar from India, or a dulcimer from Eastern Kentucky).

Humor: Try out unusual musical instruments such as spoons, a saw, or glasses of water. Laugh at your flat notes!

Early Dementia: Ask someone who can play a musical instrument to give a "concert" to the group.

Late Dementia: Music is a wonderful way to connect in late dementia. *Persons* may enjoy hearing their favorite type of music.

Sensory: Enjoy the materials that the instruments are made of (e.g., wood, metal, strings). Feel the vibrations of the notes.

Conversation: Ask for participation, "Trish, let's see how many musical instruments we can name?" Ask an opinion, "Does anyone have a favorite instrument?" Encourage discussion, "How are string instruments made?" or "How do they make the violin, viola, cello, and bass sound different?" Inquire, "Isabel, what is the difference between a violin and a fiddle?" Reminisce, "Has anyone ever played a pipe organ? Tell me about it." "Did anyone take piano lessons? Did your mother make you practice?"

An ounce of prevention...

Some people are sensitive to loud noises. Watch for signs of persons becoming anxious and agitated.

Winter Memories

Wintertime is often when things slow down. For many *persons* with dementia, this season may have been a time to be cozy at home with family. This class discussion brings the group together to enjoy all the qualities we celebrate about winter.

The Basics

Before Class: Collect information and trivia on the seasons and winter. Internet keywords include: seasons, winter, snow, snowflakes.

Collect items relating to winter, such as: winter clothing; snow globes; a sled; a toboggan; ice skates; skis; pictures of snowy landscapes; or foods that may be related to winter such as hot chocolate (regular and sugar-free), chestnuts, or a hearty vegetable soup.

At Class Time: Share the items with the group. Discuss some of the findings from your research and share winter trivia. Discuss winter memories such as sledding, sitting around an open fire, or the biggest snowfall you've ever seen. While class is in session, pass around hot chocolate for all to enjoy. If a fireplace is available, use it!

Variations: This topic can be done with any of the four seasons (see summer activity that follows).

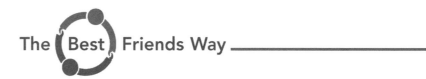

The (Best) Friends Way

Life Story: Learn about where people grew up and brainstorm how they might have experienced winter. Did anyone live in a very cold climate or a hot climate? How were winters different in each place? How did it affect the *person's* lifestyle?

The Arts: Draw a pen-and-ink sketch of a winter tree (see page 50).

Exercise: Bundle up and go outside to experience the weather. Many will enjoy the brisk air, even if it's just for a few minutes.

Humor: Joke about long-underwear or snowball fights.

Music: Celebrate winter by singing "Winter Wonderland," "Let It Snow," or "Jingle Bells."

Old Sayings: "Cold as…" See how many endings you can come up with!

Sensory: Taste a bowl of hot soup, shake snow globes, and feel the texture of warm woolen sweaters or soft fleece blankets.

Conversation: Take a survey, "Who thinks winter is the best season?" List favorite wintertime activities. Ask an opinion, "Ernie, what clothes do you associate with winter?" Play trivia, "Where in the world receives the most snowfall?" Reminisce, "Jarvis, did you ever make a snow fort?" or "Jessica, I know you grew up in Florida. How were the winters there?"

The Basics

Before Class: Collect information and trivia about the seasons and summer. Internet keywords include: seasons, summer, picnics, summer solstice, 4th of July.

Also collect items that suggest summer, such as: fly swatter, an oscillating fan; sunglasses; vintage swimsuits; suntan lotion; photographs showing summer activities such as sailing, swimming, and picnics.

Enjoy summertime foods, such as watermelon, ice cream, iced tea, and lemonade.

At Class Time: Begin by asking participants to name the first thing that comes to mind when they think of summertime. Write their ideas on a flip chart. Discuss their answers and then share the information and trivia you've learned. Reminisce about summer while looking at the summertime items. Serve food associated with summer.

Variation: Have a 4th of July party.

Summertime

In the good ole summertime! Many of us have vivid memories of summertime—which was usually a busy and fun time (although sometimes remembered for long, hot, muggy days!). Summertime activities may hold special meaning for *persons* with dementia who may recall being out of school, longer days, summer jobs, and special seasonal celebrations.

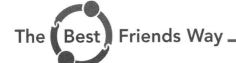

The Best Friends Way

Life Story: Think of where the *person* grew up and how this locale might affect his or her memories of summer. Did he or she chase fireflies in the country or cool down with a fire hydrant in the city? List class members' summer jobs.

Exercise: Try swimming or water aerobics classes on a warm day. Enjoy chair exercises on a screened-in porch.

Humor: Will someone confess to going skinny-dipping?

Music: Play recordings of "Those Lazy-Hazy-Crazy Days of Summer," "In the Good Ole Summertime," "In the Shade of the Old Apple Tree," "Summertime."

Old Sayings: "Dog days of summer." "Hot as… " See how many endings you can add!

Sensory: If the weather is balmy or warm, go outside and experience summer directly. Some might enjoy spitting watermelon seeds onto the grass!

Conversation: Speculate, "What are the dog days of summer?" Reminisce, "Jim, did the iceman ever come to visit? Did you catch ice chips from the back of his truck/wagon? Did anyone ever have a lemonade stand?" Discuss celebrating the 4th of July, "Juliette, did you watch fireworks and eat hot dogs? What were your summertime traditions?" List items you would take on a picnic.

An Apple a Day

Apples are a great snack and the basis for many recipes including some comfort foods. This activity is an example of how even the simplest prop, in this case apples, can be the source of a substantial activity for *persons* with dementia.

The Basics

Before Class: Gather information and trivia on apples. Internet keywords include: apples, Johnny Appleseed, specific apple varieties.

Collect as many varieties of apples as you can at the local grocery store (e.g., Granny Smith, Red Delicious, Fuji), a variety of apple corers and peelers, food made with apples (e.g., apple pancakes, apple cobbler, applesauce).

At Class Time: Discuss apples and the different types of apples. Allow the participants to taste each of the different types of apples and pick their favorite one. Have participants brainstorm all of the things you can make with apples: pie, applesauce, jelly, applejack, cider, or potpourri. Have a food made from apples ready for the group to taste.

Planning Tip: Morning or afternoon classes can prepare some goodies for *persons* to enjoy in the evening.

The 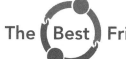 Best Friends Way

Life Story: Did anyone have an apple tree in his or her yard? Does anyone have a special recipe using apples? Was anyone a teacher who received apples from his or her students? Did anyone grow up in apple country?

Humor: Laugh about bobbing for apples.

Music: Sing "Don't Sit Under the Apple Tree with Anyone Else but Me" and "In the Shade of the Old Apple Tree."

Old Sayings: "Don't upset the apple cart." "An apple for the teacher." "Apple-polisher." "Apple of my eye."

Sensory: Taste and smell the different apples. Feel the apple peel, and hear the crunchy sound of an apple being eaten.

Spirituality: Discuss the meaning or meanings of the saying, "From a tiny apple seed grows a giving tree."

Conversation: Ask opinions, "Carrie, what do you think about these Granny Smith apples? They are too sour for me!" or "Which do you like: sweet or sour?" or "What kind of apples make the best pie?" Discuss legends surrounding apples—"Which one have you heard?" (Johnny Appleseed, William Tell, Sir Isaac Newton) Share some trivia, "Did you know that apples are 80% water?" Debate, "Do you think one bad apple really does spoil the whole bunch?"

The Basics _____

Before Class: Collect information and trivia about beans. Internet keywords include: beans, lima beans, baked beans, Jack and the Beanstalk, bean recipes.

Also collect different types of raw beans (e.g., kidney, lima, black, navy, pea, coffee) as well as various canned bean products (e.g., Boston baked beans, garbanzo beans, green beans). Consider sharing recipes using beans.

At Class Time: Share trivia and information about beans (e.g., how many products and foods come from soybeans—everything from cattle feed to plastic bags).

Prior to class, tape individual types of raw beans to index cards. During class time, pass these cards around and ask the group to guess what type of bean it is. Discuss the different uses for beans. Talk with the group about cooking beans. Taste a canned bean product.

Variations: Use a package of bean soup mix to sort and identify each type of bean.

Training Tip: Try this activity at a staff meeting to demonstrate how an activity can be built from the simplest ingredients.

The 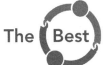 Best Friends Way _____

Life Story: Did anyone grow beans? Did anyone in the group make bean soup? What was the most common bean in the region where the *person* grew up?

The Arts: Create a colorful mosaic using different kinds of beans.

Old Sayings: "Jack & the Beanstalk." "Don't spill the beans." "Bean counter." "That doesn't amount to a hill of beans."

Sensory: Observe the smoothness and varied color of the beans. Savor the flavor of a favorite bean dish.

Spirituality: Plant some beans in a garden area and enjoy the miracle of nature as the plants grow and produce their bounty.

Conversation: Ask the following questions about beans, "What types of beans are these? What would you make with them?" Ask the *person* to teach you, "Cindi, how do you prepare beans in order to soften them enough to eat?" Learn together, "What common drink is made from a bean?" (coffee) Does chocolate come from a bean or seed?" (Chocolate is a food made from the seeds of a tropical tree called the cacao). Joke with the *person*, "I don't like lima beans, do you?" Reminisce, "Jake, did you ever read the story *Jack & the Beanstalk*?"

An ounce of prevention…

Supervise the activity carefully so the person doesn't eat the raw beans.

Colors of the Rainbow

We are surrounded by colors every day and often forget to take time to notice and enjoy them. Our life is so enriched by color—imagine if we lived in a black-and-white world! This topic brings color to life for *persons* with dementia and offers plenty of visual stimulation!

The Basics

Before Class: Collect information and trivia about rainbows. Internet keywords include: rainbow colors, pot of gold, leprechauns.

Also collect items highlighting the colors of the rainbow—red, orange, yellow, green, blue, indigo, and violet—and photos and artwork featuring rainbows.

At Class Time: Pass around and discuss the photos and artwork of rainbows. Have group members share their favorite colors. Pass around colorful items to stimulate discussion on the colors. Discuss the scientific origins of rainbows, such as what causes a double rainbow.

The (Best) Friends Way

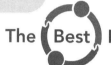

Life Story: Ask everyone about their favorite color and then use them frequently in conversation. A caregiver with knack can use even this simple piece of information in dozens of ways (e.g., noting a *person* is wearing his or her favorite color, commenting on the color of flowers, napkins, cars, and houses).

The Arts: Make a color collage by cutting pictures from a magazine that remind you of colors of the rainbow. Make a rainbow using crushed eggshells (see page 62).

Humor: "Let's look for the pot of gold at the end of this rainbow." Laugh and joke about what you would do if you found that pot of gold.

Music: Sing songs that remind *persons* of rainbow colors such as: "Blue Moon," "Yellow Rose of Texas," "Somewhere Over the Rainbow."

Old Sayings: "Black and blue," "Seeing red," see how many sayings you can come up with that involve colors.

Sensory: Enjoy the colors of the rainbow. Go outside after a rainstorm and look for rainbows! Serve and enjoy rainbow sherbert.

Conversation: Discuss how some colors have a symbolic meaning such as white for purity or purple for royalty. Engage in trivia, "What are the colors of the rainbow? Some people learned to remember them by the acronym ROY G BIV (red, orange, yellow, green, blue, indigo, and violet)." Speculate, "Joan, what if we had no color? I've heard that dogs see the world only in black and white?" Reminisce, "Fran, do you remember getting your first color television? Explore together, "What are some funny names for colors?" (fuchsia, teal, chartreuse, and mauve)

The Basics

Before Class: Collect information and trivia about hats. Internet keywords include: hats, Stetson hats, baseball caps.

Also collect various hats of all shapes and sizes: sombrero, cowboy hat, tam, top hat, ladies hat, baseball cap, and hard hat.

At Class Time: Use the information from the library or Internet to write trivia questions or to present "fun facts" during your class session.

Pass around the hats and encourage group participants to try them on. Have group participants model hats for the group. Discuss the background and uses for each of the hats. Make sure to have a camera on hand to catch all the whimsy!

The 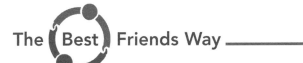 Best Friends Way

Life Story: Discuss each *person's* past use of hats. Did a woman wear hats years ago or even today? Did a man wear a hat for business attire or as part of a job (e.g., military).

The Arts: Bring in a Stetson or other cowboy hat. Go around the class asking each *person* to tell you what he or she thinks of when he or she sees a cowboy hat. Use their answers to create a group poem.

Exercise: Model the hats with a "hat parade."

Humor: Enjoy each other in the funny-looking hats!

Early Dementia: Taking pictures of *persons* in hats could be fun for someone with a flair for photography.

Music: Sing the song, "Easter Bonnet" while each *person* is trying on hats.

Old Sayings: "Hats off to you!" "Throwing your hat into the ring." "Tipping one's hat." "Wearing many hats." "Panama hats."

Sensory: Feel the texture and materials of the hats. Some may have feathers, beads, or leather.

Conversation: Speculate, "Sister Patricia, why do you think this sombrero was designed this way?" or "Why do baseball players wear hats?" Ask an opinion, "Russell, how do I look in this cowboy hat?" Reminisce, "Donna, did you ever use a hat pin? How are those used?" Discuss hat etiquette, such as men removing hats when indoors. Think together, "Why are straw hats so popular?"

Thanksgiving Blessings

Thanksgiving is a wonderful time to reminisce and think about the blessings in our lives. This can be a great topic for *persons* with dementia to remember past traditions and celebrate blessings with family and friends.

The Basics

Before Class: Collect information and trivia on Thanksgiving. Internet keywords include: turkey recipes, cranberry sauce, Thanksgiving traditions, Thanksgiving history, Plymouth Rock.

Prepare samples of food associated with Thanksgiving (e.g., cranberry sauce, turkey, stuffing, and pumpkin pie) and provide a flip chart and markers.

At Class Time: Print out information to use in trivia games or to present as "fun facts" during your class session.

Discuss Thanksgiving traditions. Share with the group the story of the first Thanksgiving. Ask the group to name things they are thankful for and write their answers on the flip chart. Taste the Thanksgiving foods you have prepared.

Variation: Note similar traditions such as Canadian Thanksgiving (the 2nd Monday in October).

The 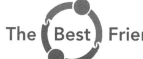 Best Friends Way

Life Story: How did the *person* celebrate Thanksgiving? What was a favorite Thanksgiving food or tradition? Has anyone traveled to Plymouth Rock where the Pilgrims landed? Did anyone hunt or raise turkeys? Who traveled to their grandparents' house for the holiday?

The Arts: Make a group collage from the written list of blessings on the flip chart. Complete a Thanksgiving Bulletin Board.

Humor: Talk about funny Thanksgiving mishaps: "We walked in to find the dog had eaten our Thanksgiving turkey!" Joke about overeating or about being "stuffed" on the turkey stuffing!

Music: Sing "We Gather Together" or "Over the River and Through the Woods"

Old Sayings: "Let us give thanks."

Sensory: Experience the tart taste of cranberry sauce, the smell of a turkey baking, and the colorful assortment of food on the table.

Spirituality: Ask if anyone would like to share something he or she is thankful for. This can create feelings of happiness and connection.

Conversation: Speculate, "Mr. Thomas, what do you think it was like to be at the first Thanksgiving?" Have a debate over whether potatoes are better than dressing or whether mincemeat pie is better than pumpkin pie. Discuss different traditions around Thanksgiving. It's a uniquely American holiday, but do other countries have a similar celebration? Debate, "Marjorie, is it called dressing or stuffing?" Discuss the best ways to make cranberry sauce.

The Basics

Before Class: Collect information related to camping. Internet keywords include: camping songs, campgrounds, camping supplies. Also collect books about camping, campgrounds, or national parks or items related to camping, such as: canteen, tent, sleeping bag, and camping pots and pans.

Obtain all of the ingredients needed to make s'mores: graham crackers, marshmallows, and chocolate candy bars.

At Class Time: Lead the group in a discussion about camping. Pass around and discuss the items related to camping. You can even pitch a tent in the middle of the group as a visual focal point. Make s'mores (in the microwave) for the group to eat while reminiscing about their camping experiences.

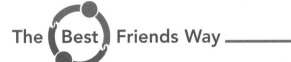

The Best Friends Way

Life Story: Do you have any campers or nature buffs in your group? Did anyone camp regularly? Did anyone live near a national park? Did anyone travel in an RV or camper? Are there any Boy or Girl Scouts in your group?

The Arts: Create a word game or puzzle using names of national parks.

Humor: Laugh about the time the tent caved in during the middle of the night or being scared by ghost stories told around the campfire!

Music: Sing old camp songs such as "Clementine."

Sensory: Knock on a canteen when it is empty and when it is full. Notice the different sounds. Explore the taste of the s'mores: crunchy graham cracker, smooth marshmallow, rich chocolate.

Spirituality: Discuss how camping out under the stars helps one feel like a part of the universe.

Conversation: Ask for help, "Martha, how do you pitch a tent? Start a fire? Cook dinner outside?" Reminisce, "Did you ever fry freshly caught fish? Did it taste better than fish bought at the store?" Discuss various national parks *persons* have visited. Ask a playful question, "How many here would like to go camping and rough it? How many would rather spend the night in a nice hotel?" Recall times sitting around a bonfire.

Camping Out

Camping is an activity many people have enjoyed at some time in their lives. It is a great opportunity to get in touch with nature. Many *persons* with dementia have camped and may have fond memories of this experience. This topic explores the experience of camping with your group.

Remembering Childhood Games

What fun it is to be a child! Many *persons* with dementia remember playing games as children and have fond memories of these games. A class activity can include reminiscing about games, playing them, or involving children in play.

The Basics

Before Class: Collect information and trivia on games. Internet keywords include: childhood games, hopscotch, red light–green light, stickball.

Brainstorm a list of as many games as you can think of: tag, kick the can, hopscotch, Mother May I?, red light-green light, pick-up sticks, or hide-and-seek. Gather together old table games such as checkers or jacks. Have a flip chart and markers ready.

At Class Time: Set games around the room to serve as cues and visual stimulation during the class time. Have the group members name games they played as children and write their answers on a flip chart. Lead the group in a discussion about their childhood games. Encourage group members to play some of the games.

Variations: Play charades (see page ??). Introduce an intergenerational aspect to the activity by inviting children to join you.

The 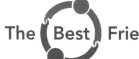 Best Friends Way

Life Story: Gather information from the life story about the *person's* childhood and the kind of games he or she played. Where did the *person* grow up—in the country or the city? Did the *person* play different games depending on where he or she lived (e.g., stickball in New York City or hockey in Canada)?

Humor: Laugh about always being "It" when playing tag.

Music: Listen to songs that became the basis for musical games: "Here We Go Round the Mulberry Bush," "London Bridge."

Old Sayings: "All work and no play make Jack a dull boy."

Old Skills: Games can involve counting, organizing, rolling dice, and shuffling cards.

Sensory: Seeing, hearing, and acting out the games are a sensory-rich experience. Be sure to pause during play and remind participants to take note of the various sensory stimuli.

Conversation: Reminisce, "What types of games did you play as a child? What was your favorite?" Ask for help, "How do you play tiddly-winks?" Ask an opinion, "George, did you play catch with your father?" Speculate, "I wonder if children today play tag and hide-and-seek like we did as children?"

The Basics

Before Class: Collect information and trivia about cities, including population figures, historical events, and famous residents. Internet keywords include: specific city names, Broadway, tallest buildings, subways.

Also collect pictures of city life taken from books or magazines and items reflecting city life: Broadway ticket stubs, major league sporting events, arts pages from newspapers and magazines, subway schedules, and maps. Have a flip chart and markers ready.

At Class Time: Create a list of big cities where *persons* have lived or visited. Discuss the cities and offer some of the information you've learned about city life from your research. Pass around your items or photographs reflecting city life to begin the discussion. Discuss major cities, and ask the group what they think of when you mention that city. Note city landmarks: New York City's Empire State Building, Seattle's Space Needle, Paris's Eiffel Tower, and the London Bridge.

Bright Lights, Big City

Many people have lived in or visited large cities. City life can be fun and entertaining. With big cities we think of skyscrapers, art museums, entertainment, shopping, and the buzz of large crowds. This topic focuses on the fun and unique aspects of big city life that many *persons* with dementia will enjoy.

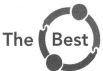

The (Best) Friends Way

Life Story: Caregivers with knack understand that many *persons* remain aware of and proud of their hometown. Focus on cities where *persons* have grown up or traveled to. Find out if he or she was a proud New Englander, Floridian, or lived in Mexico City until 18 years of age. Some *persons* enjoy it when you point out that they are a California "native" or lived in a particular city for most or all of their lives.

The Arts: Create a fabric landscape of a city skyline (see page 60).

Humor: Giggle about running into your next-door neighbor while on vacation in Paris, France.

Music: Sing or listen to "The Sidewalks of New York," "Meet Me in St. Louis," "Give My Regards to Broadway."

Old Sayings: "Bright lights, big city."

Sensory: As a class, imagine the sights, smells, and sounds of a big city zoo, ball park, or concert hall.

Conversation: Reminisce about city life experiences, "Did you shop on Michigan Avenue when you visited Chicago?" or "Have you ever traveled to the top of the Eiffel Tower?" Ask for information, "Millie, tell me about your father's grocery store on 1st Street?" Celebrate the life story, "Dan, I know you have always been an avid Yankees fan!" Share trivia, "What city has the largest population in the world?"

Celebrating Cinco de Mayo

Celebrating holidays carries on traditions of gathering together with family and friends, decorating, sharing festive foods, and singing and dancing to familiar songs.

Continuing these traditions can add interest and a feeling of happy, festive times to the lives of *persons* with dementia. Here's a sample celebration of one holiday dear to many, Cinco de Mayo, the 5th of May, Mexico's Independence Day.

The Basics

Before Class: Research the history and celebration of Cinco de Mayo on the Internet or with books. Gather together items related to the day such as: a Mexican flag, pictures of previous celebrations, mementos, music, and food.

At Class Time: Talk about the history of the day. (From this research, we discovered that Cinco de Mayo is the celebration of the Battle of Puebla in 1862 in which a small army of 4,500 Mexicans defeated an army of 6,500 French soldiers trying to gain control of Mexico. The battle stopped the invasion and was a great victory for Mexico. The day is celebrated on May 5th.)

Discuss Mexican art and culture and how it relates to the *person*. Hang a Mexican flag, look at a map of Mexico, and discuss the different regions. Create or use those decorations collected over the years and display them. Consider preparing and sharing a meal with traditional Mexican foods. Build in time for music and dancing.

Variation: Any holiday can be celebrated in a similar way.

The 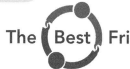 Friends Way

Life Story: Who grew up in Mexico or visited regularly? Does anyone celebrate this holiday? Who in the group likes Mexican food? Does anyone pride themselves for loving very hot and spicy food? Was anyone born on this day?

Early Dementia: *Persons* may enjoy researching holidays to plan the program using books, magazines, or even the Internet.

Music: Listen to mariachi or other Mexican music.

Sensory: Taste a cheesy enchilada or try various salsas from mild to a little spicy.

Spirituality: Many holidays have origins of a spiritual or religious nature that can be celebrated. Simply helping a *person* reflect on the special day with gratitude is spiritual and can help him or her feel connected.

Conversation: Ask *persons* from Mexico how they celebrated the holiday in their families. Discuss holidays in general, "Phoebe, do you enjoy getting ready for holidays?" Encourage diversity, "Alfonso, do you like foods from other countries?" Spend time together, "Michelle, help me set the table for tomorrow's party."

An ounce of prevention...

Celebrations may become too noisy for some persons. Be sensitive to this.

CHAPTER THREE

Let's Create

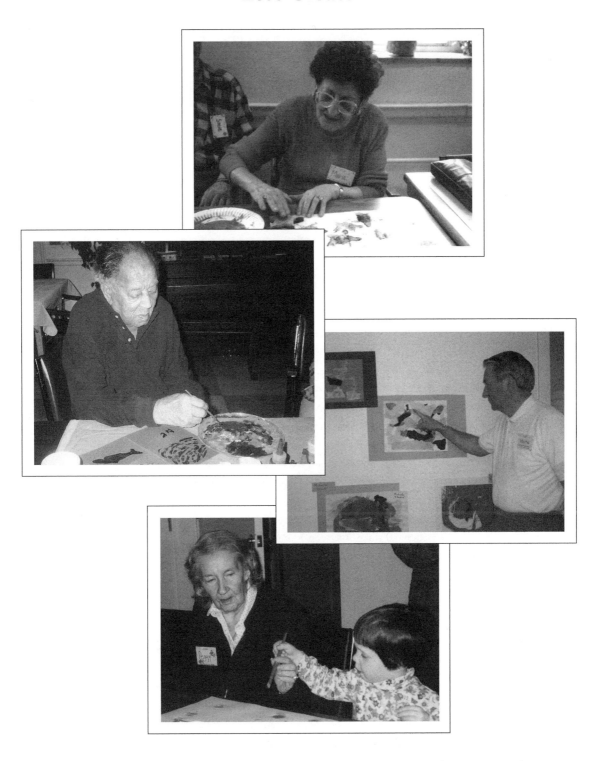

Let's Create

Many of us enjoy creative art activities whether it is painting, drawing, writing, or crafts; there are thousands of possible outlets for creative expression. These activities at their best utilize our imagination, life experiences, and strengths and abilities. They also touch the human spirit, allowing us to experience a sense of wonder and creation.

Persons with dementia continue to benefit from creative activities. Indeed some researchers feel that as cognition is stripped away by dementia, *persons* become more open to creative activities.

The goals of the activities in this chapter are to increase self-esteem, to provide a sense of belonging through socialization, to provide a new avenue for communication, to provide opportunities for *persons* to have control and make choices, and to increase positive feelings associated with making a contribution. Creative art experiences can be offered through visual art mediums, music, writing, and creative movement.

Family members or staff with knack will approach the activities suggested in this chapter by focusing on the process of creating, the doing. Art is a way of seeing. It draws emotion. Although each activity in this chapter offers the basic steps and ingredients of the project, approach the session in the spirit of the moment, let the project unfold as it will, and enjoy whatever is created.

An enthusiastic approach sets the tone for a positive art experience. *Persons* will look to you for cues as to whether or not this is something that will work. When you communicate support and encourage the *person's* efforts at creating, it will be rewarding for both of you.

Choose art activities that lend themselves to varied levels of creativity. For example, if you try the Sandpaper Art (see page 49), you may stop with one step for some, or you may add a step for those who are higher functioning. Take into consideration individual differences and interests. Adapt your approach to suit personality characteristics and personal history. What one *person* loves to do may not interest another person. Try everything.

Consider a *person's* strengths and abilities. If a *person* can cut with scissors, let him or her cut out the pictures from greeting cards. Another *person* might be good at organizing the pictures on the page. If a *person* is good with glue, let him or her glue the pictures onto your collage. If you think about what the *person* could do with the materials, then an art project may appear right before your very eyes.

Art supplies used for visual art projects should be simple, safe, easy to use, and easy to clean. Most art supplies come in non-toxic varieties. Basic supplies to have on hand for visual arts projects include paint, paper, a pair of scissors, paint brushes of many sizes, washable markers, newspapers or plastic tablecloths to cover tables, jars to hold water, white glue, pencils, pens, a ruler, and paper towels. Tempera paints are good to use for most painting experiences. Most *persons* will have success with cake watercolors as well. Scholastic grade acrylic paint may also be used if it is non-toxic.

Have lots of paper on hand. Some of the paper must be strong enough to hold paint (50–80 lb. weight). Thin paper, such as copier paper, may be used for other types of projects. For sculptures, use clay that is air-drying, non-toxic, warm, and easy to mold.

The supplies you have on hand can give you ideas. Many programs receive an abundance of donated magazines. You can also obtain free or low-cost art supplies from lumberyards (scraps, chips), newspaper printing plants (free newsprint), paint supply stores (discontinued wallpaper books), frame shops (unused mat fragments/pieces), marble/monument companies (marble and granite chips), and fabric shops (fabric and felt odds and ends).

Theme collages may be made with magazines, school glue, construction paper, a pair of scissors, and a little imagination. You may have other unusual items that people have given, such as old Christmas cards, buttons, or yarn. Create special projects using whatever supplies you have. Most small, lightweight items can be used as part of a collage (see list of collage materials on page 68).

Relax and enjoy the creative process!

CHAPTER THREE ACTIVITIES

The Basics

- Sandpaper sheets (8 x 12 inches, any grit or "texture")
- Crayons (with papers removed to make them less childish)
- Flowers or fruit to provide an image to draw

Set up the subject for drawing (e.g., flowers, fruit), and discuss the colors and lines. Use crayons to draw a picture of the subject or a creation of one's own on the rough surface of the sandpaper.

Variations: Place a piece of white paper on top of the colored sandpaper and iron with an iron set on low. Enjoy the colorful dots it creates on the paper. Another variation is to use chalk to replace the crayon. Spray the finished piece with hairspray to make the chalk drawing smudge free.

Sandpaper Art

Sandpaper art adds unusual interest to a basic still-life drawing project. The texture of the sandpaper and feel of the crayon gliding on it makes drawing a totally new experience. This can be successful even if a *person* with dementia might tell you, "I can't draw!"

The 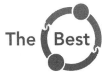 Best Friends Way

Life Story: Learn if the *person* ever worked with sandpaper in his or her work or hobbies. Does the *person* have an interest in art? Does the *person* prefer an abstract art painting or a "still life"?

Humor: "This feels like your five o'clock shadow before you shave."

Late Dementia: Accept any attempt that is made. Ask reluctant *persons* to just try out the colors of the crayon on the sandpaper. They will enjoy the feel of it whether they draw anything or not.

Music: The rhythm of soft, instrumental background music often helps the rhythm
of drawing.

Old Sayings: "Picture perfect."

Sensory: Feel the texture of the sandpaper. Smell the crayons. Discuss the colors.

Conversation: Employ some humor, "Does it give you goose bumps to touch sandpaper?" Wonder, "How is sandpaper made?" Speculate together, "Why does sandpaper come in all different textures of roughness and grit?" Encourage the *person*, "Look what a vivid color this crayon makes on sandpaper." or "Leota, would you like to try drawing with your favorite color, blue?"

Ink Paintings of Winter Trees

Winter trees form a dramatic image and symbolize the changing seasons. Without leaves, the trunk and branches become a vivid, high-contrast image. This elegant art project, featuring drawings of trees, can evoke pleasant memories and a connection to nature for *persons* with dementia.

The Basics

- White paper
- Black ink
- Fine-tip brush
- Book of trees

Demonstrate dipping the brush in the ink and painting the initial brush strokes of the winter trees. Hand the brush to the *person*. Suggest that he or she paint the tree trunk first, and then the branches of the tree.

Paint the branches to flow as the wind blows them. Paint the tree from memory or look at a real tree through the window or in a garden. You can also use books of trees to provide cues if needed.

Variations: Ask the *person* to sign his or her name using the fine-tip brush and ink or a pen. If he or she is able to do it easily, ask him or her to also write down the name of a friend or family member. Either way, framed with a colorful mat, it can make a beautiful piece of art.

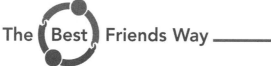

The (Best) Friends Way

Life Story: Prepare ahead by knowing the winter landscapes in the different regions where *persons* have lived. Some *persons* may have lived in the north where most of the trees are evergreen. Was the *person* an environmentalist? Did he or she live on a street named after a tree (Elm Drive, Palm Avenue).

Humor: Share happy memories of playing in a tree house or laugh about the time the fire department had to rescue a cat from a tree.

Early Dementia: Read aloud the poem "Trees," by Joyce Kilmer.

Late Dementia: Create a name drawing for these *persons*. They may find joy in recognizing their names beautifully painted in ink.

Sensory: Enjoy the smell of a pinecone or bark from a eucalyptus tree.

Spirituality: Discuss the spiritual nature of trees—the "wisdom" of an oak tree or the history of a centuries-old redwood tree.

Conversation: Reminisce, "Brad, did you ever climb a tree in winter when all the leaves were gone?" Speculate together, "What are some of the things you can see when the leaves are off the trees? A bird's nest? Mistletoe?" Ask for information, "What color is the bark on a sycamore tree?" Compliment, "Rose, that looks like a really old tree with gnarled branches. It is great!"

The Basics _____

- Paper and markers
- A dry-erase board or flip chart (so everyone can read the poem as it comes together)
- A "rhyming dictionary" (to add richness to the project)

The Process: Break the rules, as formal structure is unimportant. Pay attention instead to the flow of the words and the theme. Pick a subject (see example on next page). Decide what kind of poetry you want to write: a limerick (verse with five lines), haiku (three lines, 5-7-5 syllables), or free verse. Generate a conversation about the subject. The leader writes down key words and puts phrases together. The poem is then enjoyed as a group, with each participant receiving credit or praise for his or her participation.

Variations: Invite children to visit and read poems they are studying or ones they have written.

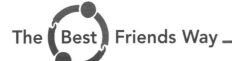

The (Best) Friends Way _____

Life Story: Was the *person* a poet or did he or she enjoy reading poetry? Did he or she learn poetry in school or memorize poems that he or she still recall today? Take some key topics from the *person's* life story or use his or her name to create a poem.

Humor: Think of funny words that rhyme such as *moose* and *goose*. Is it pronounced "pome" or "po-emm"? Read aloud a funny limerick.

Sensory: Set a poem to familiar music. Sing it or play it on the piano or guitar.

Spirituality: Read poems from *The Book of Psalms*, or other spiritual writings.

Conversation: Reminisce, "Richard, did you read nursery rhymes to your children?" Ask an opinion, "Do you think we put together a good poem?" Ask for help, "Would you read this poem for us?" Compliment, "Valerie, I love hearing you read poetry." Collaborate, "Let's try to figure out what this poem means."

Writing Poetry

This activity involves creating an individual or group poem. Poetry, as a form of expression, can have symbolic and real value for *persons* with dementia. A staff member with knack will find this to be a very powerful activity because almost everyone can contribute a word or two that, when artfully put together, creates a work of literature!

Continued on next page.

Continued from previous page.

Example: Ask a group of *persons* and the staff who are at an adult day center the following question:

What do you think about when you see a rainbow? Answer might include:

- Beautiful colors
- Peace
- Leprechauns
- Rainy day
- Pot of gold
- Red and green
- Green grass
- Cows
- Mountains
- Happy

The resulting poem might look like this:

*A rainbow is the best part of a
   rainy day.
It makes the grass green,
Which makes the cows happy!
Red and green above the
   mountains,
Leprechauns looking for a
   pot of gold.
A rainbow is beautiful colors.
A rainbow is peace.*

Freedom

I love being outside
Walking fast—I've always walked fast
Watching the birds flying high and the
   squirrels running around
Children playing and flowers blooming
   everywhere
Look at that grass, green is a good
   color for the grass and trees
Oh, how I love to walk outside
It's freedom for me.

Where I live now, sometimes she takes
   us for a walk
But its not really walking
I like to move fast, like you're on your
   way somewhere
I've had a stroke and they're afraid for
   me to walk alone
They're afraid, I'm not, but I don't
   want to cause any trouble
Being inside all the time is not good
It's not freedom for me.

Millie's Mother

She was too young to die but she
   had pneumonia
I was just a little girl, seven or eight,
   maybe
And Eva and Byron were younger
Antoinette, we called her Annie,
   and Fran were older
We all miss her—all five of us children
And father the most, he's lost without
   her
He's still sad.

But she is still young, just like she was
   when she died
With dark brown eyes and black hair
She's Italian, a Marra, from Italy
And she is beautiful, just beautiful
Still helping others in Heaven just like
   she always did
I can't wait to see her again
And father smiles when he thinks of
   seeing her.

Seeing the World

I've been everywhere
And it didn't cost me anything.
I helped them and got to see the
   world.
The children could not stay alone
While the parents worked in far away
   places.
I took care of them and
In turn we went everywhere together.

It was great fun!
You ask me what country I liked the
   best?
How can I choose one?
I loved them all, different people, all
   wonderful
I would go again if I had the chance
But before you get tied down, while
   you are young
Then you can think about it when you
   are old.

The Basics ─────────────

- White paper
- Various colors of tempera paint

Place three or four small blobs of different color paint on the paper near the center of the page. Use small plastic squeeze bottles for an easy way to apply the paint. Fold the paper in half. Smooth the paper with your hand. Open the paper and enjoy the colors and shapes you created. Experiment with the activity. You'll soon figure out the best amount of paint to apply and the colors that make the most vivid images.

Variations: "Partner Prints" is an activity two people can do together. Each *person* takes a turn applying paint to one sheet of paper. Then place another sheet of paper directly on top of the painted one and rub all four hands over it to smooth out the paint. Separate the papers and enjoy identical paintings.

Folded Paper Paintings

Everyone loves bright, beautiful colors. This activity involves applying paint to paper, then folding the paper. When the paper is then unfolded, an abstract painting is created, which evokes surprise and pleasure for *persons* with dementia.

The 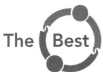 Best Friends Way ─────────────

Life Story: Did anyone ever do creative painting or paint houses? Did the *person* engage in art projects with his or her children or grandchildren? Does the final abstract design remind you of anything from the *person's* life story, such as the forest, the ocean, or even a *person's* face?

Exercise: This activity strengthens the hands and keeps the fingers nimble.

Late Dementia: *Persons* may be able to hold a paint bottle with the help of a gentle hand of an encouraging friend. If not, just look at a painting together.

Sensory: Rejoice at the beautiful colors in the finished product.

Spirituality: How does it make you feel to look at these colors? Think about the feeling of "peace." What color is it?

Conversation: Ask a humorous question, "Should we sell this to an art museum?" Speculate about the results, "Let's guess what it's going to look like when we open the page!" Ask an open-ended question, "What do you see in this picture?" Be philosophical, "Mac, you can't judge a book by its cover. Let's open up the paper and see what's inside."

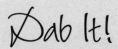 **Dab It!**

Here, an everyday item is used to create a colorful canvas. Whether painting together on a group project or working on an individual one, applying paint with small sponges allows *persons* with dementia (even those with diminished motor skills) a chance to create art.

The Basics

- Sponges (can be plain, cut into shapes on the spot, or precut)
- Tempera paint, various colors
- White or colored paper (construction paper works well)
- Small paper plate or tray to hold paint

Place a small amount of paint on the paper plate. Lay one side of the sponge flat into the paint. To keep paint off your hands, use a clothespin to grip the unpainted sides of the sponge. Dab the painted side of the sponge onto the paper a few times. The first few dabs will be darker, but continue so that your image has both light and dark sponge shapes for a nice contrast. Continue with as many different colors on one page as you choose.

Variations: Instead of sponges, dab using a balloon blown up to the size of a small apple or a potato cut in half and carved into a shape such as a flower or a heart or square. Or, use a variety of sponges such as sea sponges or cosmetic sponges.

The 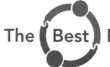 Best Friends Way

Life Story: As you do the activity, talk about elements of the *person's* life story. In a group setting, you can go around the table and comment on each class member's place of birth, special achievements, children, or occupations.

The Arts: Dab colors to make greeting cards or party invitations (see Making One-of-a-Kind Greeting Cards, page 77).

Late dementia: The balloon variation works well with *persons* with late dementia. Work with the *person* hand over hand.

Music: Think of songs that recall various colors: "Yellow Rose of Texas"; "Blue Suede Shoes"; "Blueberry Hill."

Sensory: Feel the texture of the sponge before paint is applied to it.

Conversation: Try to decide, "What do you think we should call this painting?" Joke, "Does a sponge remind you of cleaning the sink?" Share information, "Did you know that there are natural sponges that are actually sea creatures?" Give a compliment, "Arthur, the green and yellow you used make me think of spring."

The Basics ━━━━━━━━━━━━━

- Stencils, handmade (by cutting designs out of cardboard with a craft knife) or purchased at an art supply store (any kind will do if they are durable enough to hold up to paint and reuse).
- Paper
- Paint
- Small tray or paper plate to hold the paint
- Sponge or stencil brush
- Newspapers

Prepare a work area by laying out newspapers and pouring a small amount of paint into the tray. Lay the stencil over the paper. Hold the stencil still (or tape down with masking tape). Dip a sponge or brush into paint, and dab onto paper through the cutout shape in the stencil. Apply paint evenly. Remove stencil and admire your work.

Stenciling

Stenciling is not only a way to be creative with the arts, but it also serves as a practical, decorative art. If a *person* with dementia cannot draw flowers or a particular design freehand, a stencil helps him or her feel successful by creating something recognizable.

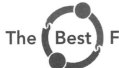 The **Best** Friends Way ━━━━━━━━━━━━━

Life Story: Did the *person* enjoy decorating his or her house or apartment? Did he or she ever paint or stencil a design on a chair or table? Select stencils that relate to the *person's* interests such as horseshoes, shamrocks, and letters or logos from a *person's* alma mater or favorite sports team. A *person's* name or initials can also be colorfully stenciled.

The Arts: Make wrapping paper by stenciling designs onto paper. Make greeting cards and invitations (see page 77) by stenciling designs onto folded construction paper or pre-made blank cards.

Humor: Laugh at some of the designs, "This looks like an elephant instead of a duck!"

Early Dementia: Invite *persons* to help create designs for stenciling.

Late Dementia: Take the *person's* hand and help him or her with the brush.

Conversation: Encourage involvement, "Let's choose a stencil to put on this card to send to your granddaughter." Provide a simple choice, "Simon, do you prefer the hummingbird stencil or the crane stencil?" or "What color would be best for this design?" Reminisce, "Did you ever make a wallpaper border by stenciling?" Ask a question about someone's native country, "Martine, is stenciling popular in France?"

Marbling

Marbling is a traditional decorative technique. It looks as if it might be difficult to do because the results are so elegant, but it is quite simple. *Persons* with dementia enjoy this activity because it is new, beautiful, and practical!

The Basics

- Cake pan (approximately 9" by 13")
- Card stock paper
- Acrylic spray paint, two or three colors
- Tongs
- Newspapers

Fill pan with water to about half full. Carefully spray the paint on top of the water in the pan, using at least two colors. (The paint will stay on top of the water). Lay the paper flat on top of the water, and lift it up with the tongs to see the marbled colors. Lay flat to dry on newspapers. Internet keywords for more information: marbling, decorative papers.

The 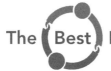 Best Friends Way

Life Story: Did the family have a marbled top dresser? Find out if the *person* enjoyed books and can recall traditional marbled covers. Most *persons* with dementia can relate to spray-painting something in their lifetime.

The Arts: Make beautiful postcards to send to friends and family out of the designs created by marbling.

Exercise: Enjoy the project outdoors and take a walk afterward.

Sensory: Bring in samples of real marble to admire the swirling designs and feel the soft surface (a kitchen designer or counter-top store may have samples or extra pieces to give away). Enjoy the unique mixture of colors and design.

Conversation: Ask an opinion, "What is the best way to paint a house?" or "Sharon, what do you see in this design?" Use humor, "Did you ever paint a room and then realize you disliked the color?" Talk about the activity, "Ron, isn't it amazing how we have ended up with something so beautiful?" Discuss the origins of the words *marbling* and *marbles*.

An ounce of prevention...

Ventilate the room by opening a window to avoid excessive fumes from the paint.

The Basics ────────────

- Paper—heavy enough to dry flat after being wet
- Tempera paint, various colors
- Drinking straws
- Wide-mouthed containers or bowls
- Liquid dishwashing detergent
- Water

Put one teaspoon water, ten teaspoons of one color paint, and one teaspoon of detergent into the bowl. Stir the mixture, and demonstrate how to blow gently until the bubbles rise above the rim of the bowl. Use knack and encourage a *person* to do something new, in this case inviting *persons* to blow into the straw. Lay the paper on top of the bowl. The colored bubbles will adhere to the page and make beautiful round designs. Continue with another color, if desired.

Variation: This is a wonderful activity to do with children; if you can, bring an intergenerational touch to your programming with this activity.

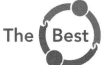

The (Best) Friends Way ────────────

Life Story: Reminisce about blowing bubbles as a child. Has anyone attended a wedding where they blew bubbles rather than throwing rice on the couple?

Humor: Laugh together, "Did you ever put too much soap in your washing machine and find the room full of bubbles?"

Late Dementia: Blow the bubbles for the *person*, and help him or her place the paper on the bowls.

Music: Sing "I'm Forever Blowing Bubbles" or "Tiny Bubbles."

Old Skills: Blowing bubbles is an old skill reminiscent of childhood.

Conversation: Observe together, "It is interesting to see so many colors inside the bubbles." Become art critics, "Do you like this modern art or do you prefer more traditional painting?" Meet a challenge together, "Mae, I think every piece of art needs a name. What should we call this painting?"

Painting with Bubbles

Blowing bubbles is a fun, nostalgic activity that can also become an art project. With this project, *persons* with dementia blow bubbles and capture them on paper for an interesting art piece.

An ounce of prevention...

Even though non-toxic materials are used, be sure to provide simple directions and supervision so the person won't use the straw as a drinking straw.

From Bell, V. (1995). Creative arts and crafts. In *Activity programming for persons with dementia: A sourcebook*. Chicago: Alzheimer's Association. Adapted by permission.

Scrap Paper Art

A torn paper project, in which pieces of torn paper are used to create various art projects, is one of the simplest and most flexible of all art activities. This activity is particularly tactile for *persons* with dementia and is interesting and colorful.

The Basics

- Construction paper in multiple colors
- White glue

Put aside a number of whole sheets of paper to use as your "canvases." Tear some construction paper into scraps of various interesting shapes, sizes, and colors. Lay out paper scraps on the background canvas. Try overlapping some of them. Use varying degrees of contrasting colors. Glue the paper scraps down.

Variations: Try using tissue paper. Crumple the paper first for an interesting texture effect. Tear out specific shapes like mountains, trees, and sun to add interest to your work. Add embellishments such as photographs, glitter, colored glue, or sequins.

The 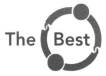 Best Friends Way

Life Story: Create a picture related to the *person's* life such as a country school house, musical notes, a sailboat, or a collage of colors reminiscent of a flower garden.

The Arts: Another option is to make simple birthday cards. Tear out shapes of a layered birthday cake, candles, and flames. Greeting cards or thank-you notes can also be created, an important motivator for *persons* who normally resist participating in art projects (see Creating One-of-a-Kind Greeting Cards, page 77).

Humor: Laugh (while ripping the paper), "This is a great way to get out our frustrations!"

Late Dementia *Persons* may be able to tear a piece of paper or press down a glued piece for it to adhere.

Old Sayings: "Waste not, want not."

Spirituality: When *persons* are free to create in their own way, they may choose to create a religious scene, which fulfills a spiritual need.

Conversation: Ask for opinions, "Do you think this piece of paper resembles a tree?" or "Do you like the dark purple?" Give a compliment, "Charlie, I like the way you put those two colors together. I wouldn't have thought of it, but it looks great!" Make a statement, "I like to use scrap paper instead of throwing it away." Encourage, "Irene, let's try something different. Let's make a picture of your new red bird house."

An ounce of prevention...

Caregivers with knack understand a person's values; a thrifty person might not want to rip a perfectly good sheet of paper. Instead, use scrap paper or tear the paper out of his or her sight.

The Basics ──────────

- A collection of odds and ends such as ribbons, feathers, buttons, jewelry, silk flowers, or anything else you can imagine! (See list of collage materials for ideas, page 68.)
- Glue or glue gun
- Poster board or cardboard

Choose one lead item that can form a base for your character (for example, a piece of driftwood that resembles an owl or a hat that can become your character's face). Add various collage materials to develop the characters.

The character can be freestanding or formed on heavy cardboard. Try to come up with a name for the character or characters created. This activity can be developed over days or weeks.

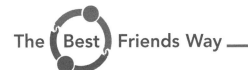

Fantasy Character Collage

At times, we all enjoy make-believe ideas, leaving our cares and concerns from the real world behind. This activity involves creating a fantasy character using collage materials. Best Friends activities involve taking chances and trying new things. *Persons* with dementia may surprise you with their interest and involvement in this fantasy creation.

The (Best) Friends Way ──────────

Life Story: Find out if the *person* ever played with puppets or perhaps put on marionette shows for his or her brothers and sisters. Has the *person* been involved in drama? Did he or she ever have a make-believe friend?

Exercise: Take a walk to find collage materials including twigs, pine cones, leaves, or other materials.

Humor: Look at a creative fantasy character and say, "That's a face only a mother could love!"

Early Dementia: Encourage a *person* to write a story involving his or her character. Read it aloud to the group.

Conversation: Begin a discussion with, "What does this look like to you?" The question is open ended. Any idea offered can be acknowledged. Use the answers to begin giving your character a personality and as inspiration for assembling the collage. Stories can develop around the make-believe characters. Work on creating a story with the group on your characters by asking questions and letting creativity soar! Reminisce about playing make believe as a child, "I used to make believe I was Superman. Wow, was that fun!"

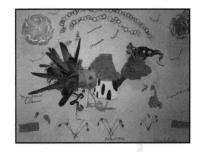

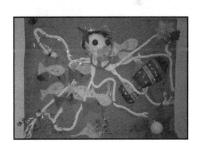

From Bell, V. (1995). Creative arts and crafts. In *Activity programming for persons with dementia: A sourcebook*. Chicago: Alzheimer's Association. Adapted by permission.

Fabric Landscapes

Landscapes are something we all admire in life and in art. Here is a simple activity in which pieces of fabric are used to create a landscape. Admiring a beautiful view is soothing and helps a *person* with dementia stretch his or her imagination.

The Basics

- Fabric scraps
- Scissors
- Heavyweight paper or card stock
- Picture books showing interesting landscapes
- White glue
- Paintbrush
- An iron

Thin the glue with a little water. Visualize your basic landscape first (for example, a wheat field, mountains, the desert). Get inspiration from real life, magazines, books, or memories. Choose fabric scraps that are consistent with the design, iron the pieces, and arrange across the paper to plan your image. Trim off any unwanted pieces.

Brush the glue on the paper and lay the fabric on top; smooth with your hands. Add drama to the picture by creating a fabric focal point for the landscape such as a tree or sun. Glue this on last.

Variations: Make fabric flowers by cutting out three large flower shapes, making each one gradually smaller than the last. Glue on the largest piece, then layer and glue the middle piece. Next, glue the smallest piece on top, and embellish with buttons glued in the center.

The 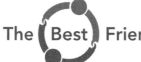 Best Friends Way

Life Story: Discuss the *person's* own interest in fabric and sewing, or ask if his or her mother was a seamstress. Reminisce about favorite trips or places *persons* have lived where there were beautiful landscapes (farms, ocean, mountains, or urban landscapes).

Music: As the group works, play music: "Blue Velvet"; "Alice Blue Gown"; "Tie a Yellow Ribbon 'round the Old Oak Tree."

Late Dementia: Feel the texture of the finished piece.

Old Skills: Choosing and arranging fabric, ironing, and cutting are all old skills.

Spirituality: Make a landscape of a sacred place such as a cathedral or a majestic mountain.

Conversation: Ask easy questions, "Misha, are you someone who prefers the city or the countryside?" or "What do you think about when spring comes around?" Present a new idea, "Jacob, what do you think about creating a seascape since you lived near the coast?" Compare, "Jane, how does this compare to making quilts?"

The Basics _____

- White glue
- Balloons
- Tempera paint
- A book or picture of the solar system
- Pie tin
- Newspaper
- Paint brushes

Talk about the planets, and show a picture of the solar system showing the planets and sun. Prepare papier-mâché paste by mixing two parts white glue and one part warm water. Stir well.

Blow up two or three balloons in different sizes to represent the planets. Tear newspaper into narrow strips about an inch wide. Cover the strips with the paste by pulling each strip through the paste mixture. Paste paper strips to balloon in many different directions until covered. Continue until four or five layers are completed. Let dry thoroughly and then paint with tempera paints.

The project can continue over a number of days or weeks until balloons representing the nine planets and the sun have been completed. Hang the planets around the sun as a mobile, or use thumbtacks and string to suspend from the ceiling.

Papier-Mâché Solar System

Since ancient times, people have gazed into the heavens and wondered about the planets. *Persons* with dementia see this activity as one of interest and intrigue.

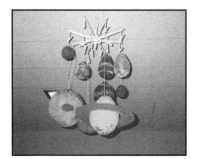

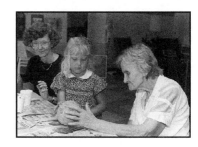

The 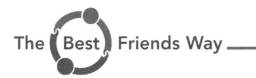 Best Friends Way _____

Life Story: Does anyone like to read science fiction stories about life on Mars? Is anyone in the group interested in astronomy or stargazing? Did anyone live away from city lights to see the stars at their brightest?

Early Dementia: This project is ambitious, and the *person* will enjoy being part of a planned effort that unfolds over a number of days and weeks.

Old Sayings: "She's starry eyed." "I'm over the moon for you." See if anyone remembers the words to the old nursery rhyme about the cow jumping over the moon ("Hey diddle diddle").

Sensory: Feel the cool, wet, sticky paste as you pull the newspaper strips through the mixture. This project requires lots of hand washing and chances for touch.

Conversation: Participants may enjoy talking about the solar system and may be able to contribute facts that they know. Discuss, "How did they name the planets?" Ask for information, "What is the difference between a star and a planet?" Daydream, "Would you like to travel to the moon?" Recall historical events such as the first shuttle mission and the first moon landing. Reminisce, "Did you ever find the man in the moon?" Ask a question, "I wonder how many planets there are in the solar system. How many do you think there are?"

From Bell, V. (1995). Creative arts and crafts. In *Activity programming for persons with dementia: A sourcebook.* Chicago: Alzheimer's Association. Adapted by permission.

Eggshell Art

This is a great activity for recyclers! Save eggshells from a month's worth of breakfasts, or ask staff and volunteers to save shells for you. Then use them to create wonderful art projects that have great texture and vivid colors. *Persons* with dementia enjoy creating art from such a familiar product.

The Basics

- Eggshells
- Rolling pin
- White glue
- Dyes (food coloring, Easter egg, or other types of dyes that are non-toxic)
- Sponges or sponge brush
- Newspapers, poster board, or heavy paper
- Containers for the dyes, one for each color

Choose a picture that has large, well-defined details (see examples on the following page). Outline the picture on a piece of poster board. The supporting material needs to be heavy enough to carry the weight of the eggshells.

Clean the eggshells by boiling them. Allow them to dry. Crush a few eggshells at a time in a heavy plastic bag using a rolling pin. Taking turns is fun. Crush until the eggshells are very fine. Decide on the colors that you want to use for each part of the picture. In small containers, add a few drops of food coloring or Easter egg dye and a splash of water. Experiment to get the color you desire.

Add crushed shells to each container, and stir until all shells are colored. Spread the shells on several sheets of newspaper to dry, keeping colors separated.

Squeeze glue around the boundary of a part of the picture that you want to color. Using a sponge or sponge brush, completely brush with glue the area to be colored. Sprinkle the shells generously over this area. Don't worry about the shells landing in various other places. Wait a few minutes and tap gently to dispose of the shells that have not been captured by the glue.

Continue working on the design, allowing one segment at a time to dry before adding additional colors. This can be an activity completed over several days or weeks.

Variations: Eggshells can be used to decorate pottery, picture frames, and ornaments.

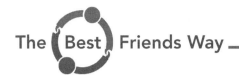

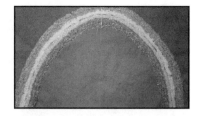

The Life Story: A *person's* life story can be portrayed in eggshell art, such as a family home, a favorite sport, climbing a tree, or bicycling.

Early Dementia: Ask the *person* to be the "Associate Director" of the project, perhaps choosing the pictures that lend themselves to eggshell art.

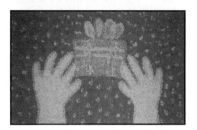

Late Dementia: *Persons* late into the disease may want to scatter the eggshells onto the glue. Eggshells may go everywhere, but the glue will catch the ones needed.

Old Sayings: "Walking on eggshells."

Old Skills: Using a rolling pin is an old skill for many.

Sensory: Running your hands through the crushed eggshells creates a distinct sensation. Also, admire the vivid colors that the eggshells pick up; they are pretty as a picture.

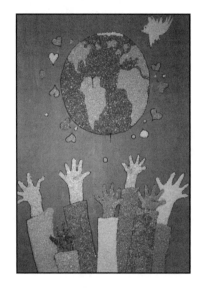

Conversation: Involve the *person*, "Michael, help me decide what color to make this boat." Ponder, "Samantha, feel these crushed eggshells. What do you think they are made of?" Reminisce, "Do these eggshells remind you of gathering up the eggs on the farm?" Compliment, "Martha, you crushed those eggshells just right."

From Bell, V. (1995). Creative arts and crafts. In *Activity programming for persons with dementia: A sourcebook.* Chicago: Alzheimer's Association. Adapted by permission.

Faux Mosaics

Mosaics are made by inlaying small pieces of variously colored material to form pictures or patterns. The dramatic contrast of a brightly colored mosaic entertains the eye and draws interest to your art program. *Persons* with dementia may enjoy practicing this ancient art technique.

The Basics

- Small (1") squares cut from paper
- Heavy paper or poster board for background canvas
- Glue

Draw a simple design on the background paper, such as piano keys or a flower. Roughly color or label the background to show where the basic colors will go. Arrange a small section of squares at a time matching the colors of the paper with your design. Glue down onto the background paper, leaving a small space between the squares.

Planning Tip: The paper squares may be cut as a separate activity ahead of time.

Variations: Cut a picture from a magazine or calendar into 1" squares, arrange on a black piece of construction paper recreating the picture and leaving a small space between the squares. Glue down.

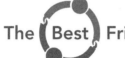

The (Best) Friends Way

Life Story: Did the *person* admire mosaics in a Turkish mosque while on vacation? Use a design to connect to the *person's* life story, such as fish for the fisherman or a guitar for the musician.

The Arts: Study ancient mosaics through books, pictures printed from the Internet, or by visiting a local museum.

Humor: When you are working on a project, use light playful conversation to entertain each other.

Late Dementia: Simply sorting the colored squares may be a satisfying activity. Alternatively, let the *person* arrange squares for you to glue down any way he or she arranges them for an interesting abstract piece.

Sensory: The spectacular mixture of colors can be visually stimulating.

Spirituality: Use a design with a spiritual motif, such as a Star of David or a cross.

Conversation: Make a connection, "Does this remind you of your bathroom tile?" Reminisce, "Have you ever seen a beautiful mosaic in a museum?" Compliment, "Nannette, I wish I had an eye for matching colors like you do!" Mull over, "I've heard that laying a tile floor with grout is difficult. Do you know anyone who has done that?"

The Basics _____

- Clay that air dries
- Thin wood board, cardboard, or a stack of old newspapers
- Wire

Warm a small piece of clay in your hands before you hand it to the *person*. Observe what the *person* does with the clay. Some *persons* may begin to shape something like a ball or a rope out of it; others may just keep molding it around in their hands. Make a positive, encouraging comment about what they do with it.

Using a ball of clay, demonstrate how to push out the middle with the thumb. Encourage the *person* to try. Continue to turn it around in your hands as you press a hole in the center to form a small pot.

Let the clay dry thoroughly (usually takes at least 24 hours). Paint the pot. Try different paint techniques such as sponge painting (see page 54) on the hardened clay.

Variations: You can sculpt abstract shapes, animals, and human figures—anything that the imagination allows. Winding long "ropes" of clay onto a clay base in a circular fashion is an easy way to make coil pots.

Make small clay tiles out of white air-drying clay (about 1" square and ¹/₂" thick). When dry, use a permanent marker to write the letters of the alphabet on each tile to use in Fun with Words (see page 100).

Clay Pinch Pots

Clay provides excellent tactile stimulation for *persons* with visual impairments or for *persons* without much finger dexterity. Clay responds dramatically to just a little pinch, so *persons* with dementia can easily see their effect on it. This activity leads to whimsical little pots you can decorate and use to store small items or as a planter.

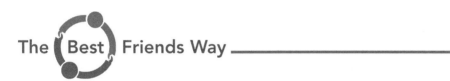

The (Best) Friends Way _____

Life Story: Did the *person* live in a part of the country where the soil was made up of clay? Did he or she, or any family member, ever throw pots?

Humor: Laugh often, "We are knee deep in mud."

Late Dementia: Involve the *person*, give plenty of eye contact, and let him or her feel the clay.

Sensory: Encourage participants to squeeze the warm, soft clay through their fingers. The next day explore the texture of the dried clay.

Spirituality: Clay is the sacred earth or mother earth. The *person* may feel a connection to nature working with clay in his or her hands.

Conversation: Speculate, "Mrs. Murdock, do you think this is what Native Americans made all their bowls out of?" or "I wonder if we can make bricks out of this clay?" Admit your feelings, "Bella, I'm having a hard time making this bowl. You seem to have it down pat." Talk about how the clay feels, "How does the clay feel to you? Is it smooth or rough? Is it cool to the touch?"

**An ounce
of prevention...**

*Provide careful
supervision to
prevent mishaps.*

Flower Pounding

This is a different way of "painting" a picture, involving very active motions. It involves transferring beautiful colors of flowers and herbs onto cloth. *Persons* with dementia enjoy the physical activity as well as the finished artwork.

The Basics

- Masking tape
- Hammer
- Unbleached muslin cloth, or cloth material pre-treated for tie-dyeing (white works best)
- Plastic cutting board or any other hard surface
- Fresh flowers and leaves (pansies, geraniums, and rose petals work well)

Place a flower, face down, onto the cloth and cover it entirely with masking tape. Turn the cloth over and place on a plastic cutting board or other hard surface that will withstand pounding. Using a hammer, pound the cloth covering the flower until the color has been absorbed into the material. Remove the tape and enjoy the colors that become a part of the cloth. If you plan to pound several different flowers onto the same cloth mark with tape the side for pounding.

Planning Tip: If the cloth is not readily available, watercolor paper can be used.

Variations: You can outline the flowers with a permanent marker for a finished look. Hangings, pictures, place mats, napkins, and quilt squares are some of the finished products that you can make from this activity.

The 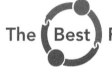 Best Friends Way

Life Story: Look for *persons* who enjoy being actively involved. Many *persons* have used a hammer in routine fix-it projects or as a career. Does the *person* have a favorite flower? Use the *person's* favorite color.

The Arts: Arrange a display of the finished pieces, and enjoy the surprised look of others when you explain how they were created.

Humor: Use humorous language, "Just give me a hammer and there goes my thumb!"

Early Dementia: *Persons* in early dementia can lead a small group, helping others choose flowers, taping their flowers to the material or paper, and showing others how to begin.

Old Skills: The old skill of pounding can release pent-up energy.

Sensory: The flowers transfer beautiful colors onto the cloth or paper. Feeling the cloth and flowers is stimulating to the senses.

Conversation: Encourage, "Take this hammer and pound right here on top of this flower." Excite the senses, "Eve, look at this beautiful purple flower. Let's smell it." Generate ideas by asking, "I wonder how these vivid colors come from a tiny seed?" Ask an opinion, "Florence, I like this pansy best. Which of these two flowers do you like the best?" Reminisce, "I'll bet you used a hammer often when you worked on that horse farm fixing all those long white fences."

The Basics _____

- A box large enough for a piece of paper (8½" by 11") to lay down flat inside. Cut the sides of the box down to approximately 3" tall
- Masking tape
- White paper
- Tempera paint
- A few marbles
- A few plastic spoons
- Small containers for paint

Tape down the paper onto the bottom of the box. Place paint in the small containers, a different color for each container. Place one marble in each container of paint. Using the plastic spoon, move the marble from the container and place it in the box. Roll the box around causing the painted marble to color the page. Take the first marble out of the box and put in another marble of a different color. Repeat the routine with as many colors as desired.

Painting with Marbles

Marbles have been found in ancient ruins and they are still popular today as game pieces, decorative accents, and collector's items. Here is another way to make marbles useful. *Persons* with dementia will have lots of fun working with their old friend, the marble, to create beautiful abstract art.

The 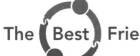 Best Friends Way _____

Life Story: Find out who played marbles as a child—maybe at school, at recess, or before or after school. Does anyone remember losing marbles as a result of losing the game? Does anyone still have his or her childhood marble collection?

The Arts: Make your own marbles for this project out of clay. (see page 65)

Humor: Joke, "This is the easiest art lesson that I have ever had."

Late Dementia: The *person* may be able to hold the box and gently tip it to move the marble around. Other hands can assist as needed.

Music: Play background music as you move the marbles around and around.

Sensory: Feel the smooth, hard glass of the marble. See the swirl of colors, and the way the light reflects off the marble.

Conversation: Think together, "Robin, I have heard of a cat's-eye marble. Do you know what one looks like?" Ask for clarification, "Did just boys play marbles or did the girls like to play, too?" Reminisce, "Do you remember playing Chinese checkers? That game was played with marbles, too." Engage a *person* who is reluctant to participate, "Grace, let's hold this box and move the marble around together."

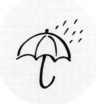

An ounce of prevention...

Be vigilant. Keep up with the marbles. They resemble hard candy.

Collage

Collage is one of the most flexible art projects. It is ideal for *persons* with dementia because *persons* can explore the materials and anything goes. Enjoy the different materials and let the creativity flow.

The Basics

- Heavy paper, cardboard, or poster board for background
- Plain white glue or glue gun
- Miscellaneous small items (see collage materials list below).

Collages can be based on any subject or a collection of interesting items. Ask open-ended questions to include the *person's* preferences such as, "What do you think about starting with some of these pretty flowers?"

Glue the first item to the cardboard. Continue adding items chosen by the group.

Variations: Collages may be based on a subject, a holiday, or a color. Build up for a collage sculpture. Collages may be made with other themes, such as a picture collage, a word collage, a fantasy collage (see Fantasy Character Collage, page 59), or a postcard collage (see page 181).

Collage Materials

Almost anything can be used for a collage as long as it is clean and lightweight (so it can be easily glued to the background).

aluminum foil	junk mail	plastic spoons
beads	keys	postcards
bells	lace	puzzle pieces
bottle tops	leaves	ribbon
broken jewelry	magazines	sequins
broken toys	make-up brushes	shells
bubble wrap	meat trays	shoelaces
business cards	nuts & bolts	silk flowers
chewing gum wrappers	nutshells	small gift boxes
clothes pins	old art projects	small milk cartons
coffee filters	old buttons	sponges
colored paper	old calendars	stickers
corks	old cards	sticks
cotton balls	old compact discs	stones
dried beans	old movie tickets	tags
dried flowers	old phone book pages	travel brochures
egg cartons	old stamps	tree bark
eggshells	paper doilies	twine
empty ribbon holders	pencils	used envelopes
feathers	photographs	used gift wrap
greeting cards	picture frames	wallpaper
ice pop sticks	pieces of wire screen	wire
jar lids	pipe cleaners	yarn

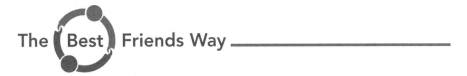

Life Story: Make positive references to a *person's* history, "Charles, you have excellent organizational skills demonstrated by your successful dry cleaning business. Will you lend us a hand with this project?"

Humor: Laugh about having everything in the collage but the kitchen sink.

Early Dementia: Some *persons* will delight in having the freedom to create their own design from start to finish. Remember the finished product is whatever the *person* comes up with.

Late Dementia: Gently encourage the *person* to participate at any level that feels comfortable.

Sensory: Collage projects encourage tactile stimulation and other sensory possibilities. Sometimes a *person* will like to touch and hold an interesting object found in the collage box.

Conversation: Say what the colors and shapes remind you of. Name the collage and enjoy safe, easy conversations about it. Ask opinions, "Do you think we should add something bright in color along the side over here?" Share an idea, "This reminds me of planning a garden. What does it remind you of?" Reflect, "I wonder where Jane got this sack full of things for us to use. Do you save everything like Jane does?" Compliment, "I can tell that you like jewelry. You have jewels hanging from all the tree branches. It looks magical."

Handmade Paper

Handmade paper is an elegant way to use recycled materials and learn something new. Most *persons* with dementia have never tried doing this activity and appreciate the novelty of a new experience when supported by a caring staff member or friend.

The Basics

- Paper scraps (should not be glossy, coated, or newsprint)
- A mould (a frame with screen attached) and a deckle (a frame without a screen) that can be purchased as part of a papermaking kit sold in craft stores. An 8" x 10" picture frames without the glass can be used. Stretch window screen over opening and staple around back edges to make the mould.
- A container or tub large enough to hold the mould and deckle
- A blender
- Old towels
- Laundry starch
- Bucket of water
- A mug to transfer water

Prepare the materials: tear paper scraps into pieces that are roughly 1" square. Fill blender about one third full with the paper pieces. Add water to fill blender to about two-thirds full. Blend 3 seconds to make a "pulp slurry."

Pour mixture into the tub. Continue to do this step until the slurry is about 4" deep. Add 1 tablespoon of dry or liquid laundry starch. Hold the mould with the screen side up and place the deckle on top of the mould. Hold the mould and deckle together, and dip into the tub of slurry, tipping up one end of the mould and deckle, gently lifting out of the water to scoop up slurry and let water drain through the screen. The deckle will catch and form the slurry on top of the screen. Repeat the dipping step two or three times until you have an even layer of slurry on top of the screen, inside the deckle.

Take the deckle off and turn the mould carefully upside down on a thick stack of newspapers.

Blot the excess water up with towels through the screen. Carefully separate the mould from the new sheet of paper and lay on a stack of newspapers. If it is too wet, it will tear when you try to remove the paper from the mould. If this happens, blot off more water. The paper will dry in approximately 12–24 hours.

Variations: Add bits of herb leaves or tiny flower petals.

The (Best) Friends Way _____

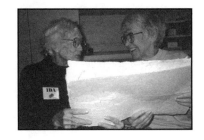

Life Story: Did anyone work for a newspaper? Did the *person* have professional letterhead or embossed stationary? Did someone maintain a long correspondence with a pen pal or send hand-written notes to friends and families?

The Arts: Handmade paper has a utilitarian purpose but also is an art in itself. Frame the paper as a work of art.

Old Skills: Blotting the water with the towels is an old skill from house cleaning.

Sensory: Putting hands in the slurry will splash a little bit. Enjoy the playful time!

Spirituality: Carrying on a centuries-old tradition can be can help a *person* feel like part of something much larger than him- or herself.

Conversation: Learn something new, "Did you know that the first paper was made in Japan in 1600?" Appreciate your work, "I think it feels good to make something new out of something that would otherwise be thrown away? I think we are helping our planet by saving a tree." Plan ahead, "Jeremy, it will be good to have this stationery done so we will have a ready supply of thank-you notes."

CHAPTER FOUR

Doing for Others

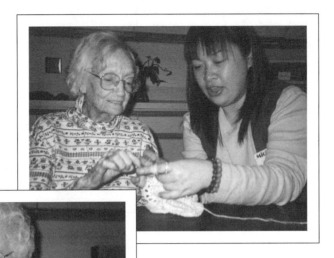

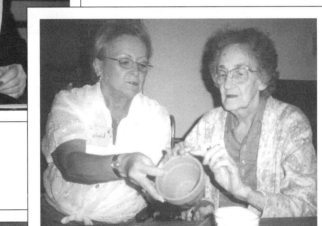

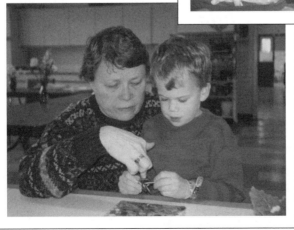

Doing for Others

Most of us receive satisfaction from helping our friends, neighbors, family members, or community at large. The same is true for *persons* with dementia. At an early-stage support group attended by one of the authors, one man commented, "I want to feel productive, like I can still do something to help others." This chapter consists of activities designed to address his need and the need of many others with dementia. Whether it is creating a gift for a grandchild, teaching someone an old skill, helping wildlife during a particularly snowy winter, giving someone a romantic Valentine, or mentoring and supporting young children, *persons* with dementia have much to give and want to make a difference in the lives of others.

From a caregiver's perspective, this chapter is important because it provides a tool to encourage cooperation. When a *person* with dementia is asked to do something, a common answer is "No." He or she may not understand what you want, may have trouble initiating new things, or simply may not see the value in that activity. When a caregiver employs knack and suggests that an activity will help others, old social graces are evoked. The ideas in this chapter can turn a "no" into a "yes."

One example is *Bead Work* (see page 82). A man with dementia may never have tried something like this or never have had an interest in jewelry making. Suggesting that he make the beads as a gift for another (perhaps his wife, sister, or daughter) can motivate him to jump right in. He can then not only experience the joy of the activity but also the pleasure of giving a gift and receiving praise and thanks for his efforts.

It is important to teach staff to reframe an activity for a *person* who is resistant as "helping" or "doing for others." For example, a staff member at an assisted living community might ask a *person* to attend an exercise class. The *person* may or may not agree to the staff member's request. Yet if the staff member asks the *person* for help arranging the chairs or help in leading the exercises, the dynamic might be quite different with the *person* readily agreeing to help.

Best Friends activities encourage thinking outside the box, taking chances, and trying new and different things. Thus not all of the activities in this chapter revolve around creating objects—many are more experiential such as *Planning an Art Show* (page 90). These ambitious activities allow a *person* to feel a part of daily life and see the fruits of his or her labor.

Volunteering would have been considered an outrageous suggestion for a dementia activity book a few years ago, but we now know that some *persons*—with assistance and modifications—can maintain volunteer work or take on new projects (e.g., helping with a newsletter mailing). Nothing ventured, nothing gained.

A successful activity program not only provides creative and rich experiences for *persons* with dementia but also helps a staff member or family member develop knack, the art of doing difficult things with ease. Learning how to reframe many requests as "helping" and recognizing a *person's* basic altruism are powerful tools that can be applied in all aspects of dementia care.

CHAPTER FOUR ACTIVITIES

The Basics ────────────

- Card stock or other heavy paper
- Watercolors
- Magic markers
- Tempera paint and brushes
- Other decorative material, such as cloth; felt; torn paper; dried flowers, leaves, or grasses; recycled artwork and greeting cards; and pictures from magazines

Start by showing the group a commercial greeting card or one that has been made by hand. Then, have each person make his or her own card, decorating any way they like.

An easy way to make the card is to fold an 8¹/₂" by 11" sheet of paper or card stock in half, cut into two sheets and fold each half sheet. Alternatively, the sheet can be folded in fourths to eliminate the cutting. Decorate the card using some of the materials listed above.

Variations: Invitations, bookmarks, and picture frames can be made using this method.

Creating One-of-a-Kind Greeting Cards

Greeting cards, marking life's special occasions and milestones, help us keep in touch with friends and family. *Persons* with dementia often understand and appreciate the significance of these cards. This activity results in individualized, handmade greeting cards.

The 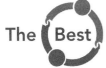 Best Friends Way ────────────

Life Story: Did the *person* regularly send cards for a birthday, special occasion, or no occasion at all? You might discover that the *person* worked in a drug store that sold cards. Use lyrics from the *person's* favorite song or words from his or her favorite poem as part of the card.

Humor: Joke about humorous cards that say, "Sorry I missed your birthday. Does it fall on the same day each year?"

Early Dementia: Encourage the *person* to write a message on the card to friends or family. Making cards for others and discussing them can be a conduit for sharing feelings or an emotional release, preventing pent-up frustration, sadness, or grief.

Old Skills: Take advantage of old skills of cutting, pasting, folding, and drawing. Have the *person* help place postage stamps on cards that you are mailing.

Spirituality: Religious motifs or scenes from the arts or from nature can be incorporated into cards. Use cards to recognize and celebrate spiritual holidays.

Conversation: Compliment, "I like the way you trimmed that picture to fit the cover of the card." Reminisce, "Did you send postcards to your friends when you were young?" Ask an opinion, "Miss Alyce, do you think this design is too big for this card?" Work together, "Let's use a lot of bright colors for this Kwanzaa card." Tease, "You slapped that paint on just like you did when you painted that barn!"

Making Envelopes for Greeting Cards

Who hasn't looked for an envelope to fit a particular card or to mail a letter? Creating tailor-made envelopes is an activity that *persons* with dementia and caregivers enjoy because the result has so many practical applications.

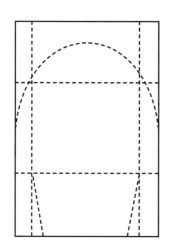

The Basics

- Sheets of 8½" by 11" paper (any color)
- Ruler
- Scissors
- Glue

Draw a line 3¼ inches from the bottom and from the top of the paper. Fold and unfold along each line to create a crease. Draw a line one inch from the left and right side of the paper. Cut these inch-wide strips off except from the middle section of the paper. Round the top section for the flap of the envelope. Taper the bottom section slightly. Leave half of the 1-inch strip nearest the bottom of the middle section intact, and taper the other half to the upper corner of the middle section. Fold the sides into the middle and put glue on the surface facing up. Fold the bottom flap up and adhere it to the side section (see diagram).

Variations: Cards and envelopes can be sold, individually or in packets. It is fun for the group to have a project that makes money for the program or as a community fundraiser. Use colorful pages from magazines to make a particularly vivid envelope.

The 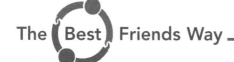 Best Friends Way

Life Story: *Persons* may have been mail carriers, worked in a post office, or stuffed envelopes as a secretary or volunteer.

The Arts: Decorate the envelope with stamped designs.

Early Dementia: The *person* can create his or her own personal stationary or be in charge of the fundraising effort if envelopes are sold.

Old Skills: Measuring, cutting, and folding are old skills.

Conversation: Explore history, "What do you know about the Pony Express?" Encourage, "Yes, just cut along that line. That's great." Compliment, "You have a good eye for measuring and folding. You are now in charge of that department." Ask opinions, "Juan, which color envelope do you think will look best with this card?" Have fun, "I like this one so much. I think I will send it to myself!" Discuss, "How many days do you think it will take this letter to get to Chicago?" Do you think the post office does a good job?"

The Basics

Before class, precut the following pieces of wood, ³/₄" thick:
- Tower: back piece (3¹/₂" by 11¹/₄"); front piece (3¹/₂" by 9");
  two side pieces (2¹/₂" by 10¹/₂"); top piece (3¹/₄" by 3¹/₂")
- Base: one piece (7³/₄" by 5"). Feeder tray pieces (7"),
  and two side pieces (5") and half round (³/₄")
- Hardware: eight #4 (1¹/₂") nails; twelve #6 flathead (1¹/₂") screws;
  and four #4 flathead (¹/₂") screws
- Hanger: Chain (10"); two screw eyes (¹/₂"); hinge (¹/₂" by 1¹/₂")
- Can of marine varnish (small)
- Hammer, screwdriver, and paintbrush

Screw back piece to side pieces, with back piece extending ¹/₂"
at the top. Screw front piece to sides, level at top. Use four #4
screws and hinge to attach top. Screw feeder tower to back of base.
Nail the ³/₄" half rounds to sides and front of base to form the feeder
tray. Attach the chain with screw eyes. Apply two coats of varnish,
let dry thoroughly.

Planning Tip: If this project proves too daunting, there are many
easy-to-assemble birdhouse kits available.

Variations: A very simple bird feeder can be made from filling
pinecones with peanut butter and rolling them in birdseed.

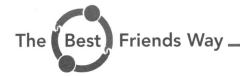

The (Best) Friends Way

Life Story: Use the life story to find out if any participant in the activity has been a
carpenter, someone who fed birds in the park, or a member of the Audubon Society.
Some individuals are passionate about bird watching as a hobby.

Early Dementia: This is a somewhat complex activity that may appeal to a *person*
with early dementia, particularly if he or she likes carpentry or is mechanically
inclined.

Old Skills: There is an old skill for most everyone—hammering, screwing, sanding, painting, and measuring.

Conversation: Reminisce, "Ellie, did you ever feed pigeons in Central Park when
you lived in New York?" Ask advice, "Do you think this needs another coat of varnish?" Enjoy doing for others, "Do you think your grandson will enjoy this for his
birthday?" Ask for information, "Where can we find out what type of seeds are
best for the birds in our area?" Take out a field guide to birds and discuss different
species; try to identify and catalog your visitors to the feeder.

Making Bird Feeders

Watching birds at a feeder can
give us hours of enjoyment during
the course of a week. *Persons
with dementia take delight from
watching their fine feathered (best)
friends and from the satisfaction of
creating a feeder for them to use.
Here is a do-it-yourself recipe for
a bird feeder.*

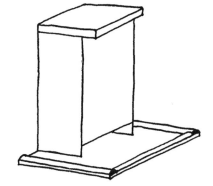

An ounce
of prevention...

*Provide extra supervision
when doing projects like
this, which feature sharp
or heavy tools.*

From Bell, V. (1995). Creative arts and crafts. In *Activity programming for persons with dementia: A sourcebook.*
Chicago: Alzheimer's Association. Adapted by permission.

Creating Wrapping Paper

Holiday time or special occasions, such as birthdays, are fun times to wrap gifts in colorful paper. *Persons* with dementia have been a part of this celebrative time and with some assistance can capture the excitement of preparing for a holiday or special event.

The Basics

- White tissue paper
- Food coloring or Easter egg dyes
- Containers for the color mixtures

Begin by showing a finished sample. Then, help participants to fold a sheet of tissue paper until it is about a 3-inch square. It can be folded any way a *person* wants to fold it. Put colors (food coloring or Easter egg dyes) in small containers. Add a small amount of water. Dip corners of the folded paper in the same or different colors making sure to just get the corner wet. Let dry completely. Don't worry if the colors blend together. It just makes the wrapping paper more interesting. When the paper is thoroughly dry unfold it to use as wrapping paper.

Variations: Plain brown paper can be decorated with markers, paints, or stamping to make attractive wrapping paper. Use a digital camera and color printer to print photos on labels or stickers to put on the gift-wrapping paper. Caregivers with knack understand that *persons* often retain a need to help others and be productive; ask them for help wrapping birthday, wedding, or holiday presents.

The 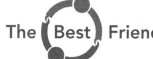 Best Friends Way

Life Story: Did a *person* gift-wrap purchases when he or she worked at Macy's department store? Did he or she work on a holiday fundraiser gift-wrapping presents at the mall? How many *persons* did all the family gift wrapping?

The Arts: Fold the colored paper to make fans to use for decoration.

Humor: Be amused about the way presents are opened. Find out if the *person* carefully unwraps a present to save the paper and bows or tears the present open impatiently.

Old Sayings: "I'm all thumbs." "The gift without the giver is bare."

Spirituality: Discuss the meaning of the saying, "It is better to give than to receive."

Conversation: Encourage by saying, "Let's dip this corner of the paper into this pretty blue color." Ask an opinion, "What are the best colors to use for wrapping wedding presents?" Joke, "Eva, I think I need three hands to wrap this present." Reminisce, "Did you open your presents on Christmas Eve or Christmas Day?"

The Basics

- Colored tissue paper
- Recycled artwork or pictures from magazines
- Glue
- Small paint brushes
- Small tray to hold water
- Clay flower pots, vases, or plastic eggs

Tear the tissue paper into small pieces. Mix the glue with a small amount of water. Brush the surface of the article (flower pot, vase, etc.) with the glue mixture, just a small area at a time. Press pieces of paper onto the object, over the glue. Continue until the surface is completely covered with different colors of paper. Then brush the entire article with a coat of the glue to waterproof it. A black marker can be used when the project is completely dry to outline the colors to make it look like stained glass.

Planning Tip: Search the Internet for the interesting history behind this centuries-old artform.

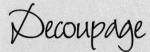

Decoupage is the technique of applying paper onto a smooth, hard surface with a brushed-on glue coating. *Persons* with dementia often enjoy this colorful and easy way of decorating. This activity results in a hand-decorated container to give as a gift.

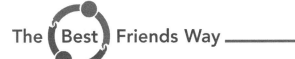

The Best Friends Way

Life Story: Travel magazines from a *person's* home state—for example *Sunset Magazine* (west coast), *Southern Living*, *Yankee* (New England), or magazines involving special interests of the *person* (cats, horses) can be used to create an individualized activity. Decoupage a picture frame with family snapshots.

Exercise: Fine motor movements of the hand are enhanced by this activity.

Late Dementia: Invite *persons* to choose a color. Help them by taking their hand in yours and placing a piece on the object (do this only if the *persons* seem interested).

Sensory: Comment on the colors and what colors go well together. Ask for opinions and decisions about what colors to use and where to place them. Let the *person* handle the finished pots, vases, or other articles.

Conversation: Celebrate a job well done, "Patrick, these clay pots look much better now. Just look at what we did to spruce them up!" Give a *person* a challenge by saying, "This is called decoupage. I wonder how you spell that big word?" Reinforce the joy of doing for others, "Delores, these Easter eggs will be fun for the children to find on their hunt next week." Compliment, "You have used such pretty colors." Speculate, "Dorothy, you enjoy language. Decoupage is a French word. I wonder what it means?"

Bead Work

Bead work is an ancient art. Making jewelry from beads to give as a gift can be a creative and satisfying activity for *persons* with dementia who will enjoy the process as well as the final outcome.

The Basics

- Beads in different shapes, colors, and sizes
- Wire for stringing

Sort the beads first, asking *persons* to help. Have a necklace or bracelet already made as an example. Give each person an opportunity to choose between a necklace or a bracelet. Start stringing beads in a pattern right away. Some will need help to begin.

The 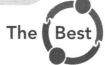 Best Friends Way

Life Story: Discover if a *person* enjoyed bead work in jewelry, purses, or on a party gown or wedding dress. Has anyone lived or visited in the southwest and seen the Native American crafts with intricate bead work?

Early Dementia: This activity can be as complex and creative as a *person's* functional level allows. Intricate patterns can be designed.

Late Dementia: The sights and sounds of the group working at a task can help prevent isolation.

Old Skills: The skill of threading is a familiar one and can be done easily by *persons* with good manual dexterity.

Sensory: The feel of the beads, different shapes, textures, and the vivid colors are stimulating to the senses.

Spirituality: Beads have meaning in some religious practices (e.g., rosaries and prayer beads).

Conversation: Reminisce, "Leticia, did you wear lots of jewelry when you were a little girl? What kind of jewelry do men wear? Did they wear cuff links? Tie pins? Watch fobs?" Chit-chat, "What do you call this color? Is it pink or rose? Is this one navy blue or aqua?" Ask advice, "Would you put these two colors together?" Give a choice, "Do you like bright red beads or dark green beads?" Compliment, "Those colors are beautiful together. Your granddaughter will love the bracelet that you have made for her."

An ounce of prevention...

Be cautious if a person tends to put objects in his or her mouth. . . It's okay if the person wants to keep the finished product— some of the best gifts are gifts we give ourselves.

The Basics

Look for opportunities for *persons* with dementia and children to be together. These can include art projects and music time; indoor bowling, basketball, ring toss, and other indoor games; working simple educational puzzles; cooking and baking; flying kites and taking walks; worshipping together; and reading aloud to preschool children.

Consider forming a partnership with a specific school or schools. Many schools are involved in community service or have an "adopt a grandparent" program.

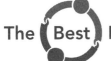 The (Best) Friends Way ──────────

Life Story: Compare names of the children and residents. Look for common birthdays and hometowns. *Persons* may have worked professionally with children in child care centers or as teachers and many are parents and grandparents themselves.

Exercise: A *person* can toss a ball with a child or take a walk together.

Late Dementia: *Persons* may enjoy holding a baby or having a baby held close to them to caress and admire.

Music: Sing songs familiar to both groups such as Christmas carols or lullabies.

Old Sayings: There are countless nursery rhymes and stories that can be shared with children. Encourage *persons* to read to children and vice versa.

Sensory: Watching children at play and hearing their laughter provide rich sensory stimulation.

Spirituality: Children represent new life, bringing hope for the future.

Conversation: Reminiscing can revolve around raising children by asking for an opinion, "Should they be seen and not heard? Do children dress differently and act more grown up today?" Talk about how good it feels to be able to make a difference in a child's life after saying, "You taught Myron how to fish. You made him very happy." Compliment, "All children seem to love you!"

Sharing Life with Young Children

Children allow us to be young again, to cut loose, have fun, be creative, and even be silly. Small children give unconditional love and generally accept the cognitive losses of *persons* with dementia without concern.

An ounce of prevention...

Sometimes the energy and noise of children can be stressful to persons; *consider keeping the time together short.*

Potpourri

Many people remember gathering and drying flower petals to give their homes and especially their closets a sweet aroma long before commercial air fresheners were available. More recently, potpourri has been a popular gift item. *Persons* with dementia may enjoy creating potpourri to keep for themselves and to give to others.

The Basics

- Flower petals and herbs
- Scented oil to refresh the potpourri
- Containers for packaging gifts (plastic bags, paper sacks, or small baskets)

Have some potpourri already made to show to the group. Pluck the petals of flowers or the leaves of herbs (fresh or those that are ready to be discarded). Spread the petals and herbs out on newspaper to dry. This can be a fulfilling activity in itself.

When the petals and herbs are thoroughly dry, add a few drops of scented oil (optional) and mix thoroughly. Package in paper sacks, plastic bags, or small baskets.

Variations: Fill small sachet bags with potpourri for special gifts for friends and family.

The 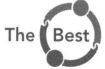 Best Friends Way

Life Story: Consider whether the *person* was interested in home décor and would have taken time to display a bowl of potpourri. Did the *person* have an herb garden or cook with herbs? Did the *person* have a rose garden and collect rose petals for various projects?

The Arts: Decorate the paper bags filled with the potpourri (see Stenciling, page 55).

Exercise: Collect herbs and flowers from outdoor gardens.

Old Sayings: Pluck the petals of a daisy while saying, "He loves me, he loves me not."

Sensory: Smell the aroma of the herbs and flowers, and touch the flower petals. See the amazing colors of red, yellow, orange, lavender, and blue. Hear the voices of people working together. If you use scented oil, pass it around for everyone to smell.

Conversation: Reminisce, "What were the names of some perfumes of long ago? Was there one named 'Lily of the Valley' and one named 'Evening in Paris'? Did you ever wear Chanel Number 5?" Have fun, "Did your boyfriend ever wear cologne?" Offer choices, "Which basket do you want to fill with potpourri, this little white one or this blue one?" Share your feelings, "Laura, your children will be so pleased with these beautiful gifts!"

An ounce of prevention...

Before beginning this activity, check to ensure that none of the participants are allergic to flowers or herbs.

The Basics

- Red and white sheets of paper or card stock
- Paints
- Markers
- Lace or paper doilies
- Magazines
- Scissors, paste, stapler
- Pens or pencils

Have some completed Valentines available as examples. Encourage the *person* to cut out a variety of sizes of paper hearts. Assemble materials that you will use to decorate with the Valentines on the table. Talk about making a Valentine for someone. Some *persons* will have their own ideas for a design. Others need help to get started. Some will want to watch for a while.

Variations: Have fun making Valentines with verses using pictures of fruits and vegetables from seed catalogs: "My heart (BEETS) for you"; "Do you (CARROT) all for me?"; "You are the (APPLE) of my eye"; "(PEAS) be my Valentine."

Be My Valentine

Can you remember giving your first Valentine? Valentine's Day has been observed for centuries. Many *persons* with dementia will relate to the giving and receiving of Valentines and to celebrating this memorable holiday!

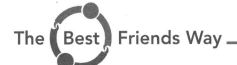

The (Best) Friends Way

Life Story: Discuss different traditions of Valentine's Day, and note that some cultures/societies do not celebrate this holiday. Is someone in the group gifted with writing poetic verse? Did anyone make homemade Valentines to give to classmates? What is the name of the *person's* spouse or partner? Remember a first kiss.

The Arts: Using the words on candy "conversation" hearts, create poems.

Humor: Tease about a girlfriend/boyfriend. "Did you kiss your sweetheart on the first date?"

Music: "Let Me Call You Sweetheart" "My Funny Valentine"

Old Sayings: There are many sayings associated with love and Valentine's Day, such as "Roses are red, violets are blue, sugar is sweet, and so are you!"

Sensory: Conduct a chocolate tasting!

Conversation: Reminisce, "Did you have a Valentine Box at school?" Speculate, "I wonder how Valentine's Day got started?" Give a choice, "What color do you want for your Valentine, red or white?" Provide an opportunity for an opinion, "What do you think about the size of this heart? Is it too big?" Tease, "Let's use this fancy lace. It looks like you."

An ounce of prevention...

If someone is sad thinking about a past friend or loved one who has died, or has other emotions surrounding the holiday, be sure to give that person some individual attention and time to express him- or herself.

Sock Monkeys

This activity involves making a classic toy that is familiar to many people: a stuffed monkey from socks. *Persons* with dementia relate to this nostalgic toy and retain their interest in doing for others, especially for children.

The Basics

- Pair of Original Rockford Red Heel socks purchased locally or ordered from Fox River Mills, Inc., Osage, Iowa 50461 (instructions for making stuffed monkey are inside the package)
- Nylon hosiery or cotton batting for stuffing
- Black and white thread and sewing needle
- Small black buttons

To make the body, turn the first sock inside out. Sew a $1/2$" seam on both sides of the center of the sock, starting 3" from the white heel and going across the end of the top. Cut the sock between the seams and to within $1 1/2$" of the white heel. This leaves an opening in the crotch. Then, turn the sock so the seams are inside and use the crotch opening to stuff head, body and legs; stitch this opening closed.

With the second sock, the *person* will create the arms, mouth, tail, and ears. For the arms, cut the upper part of the other sock into two pieces. Seam, rounding the ends and stuff the arms.

For the mouth, cut the heel from the sock, leaving a brown edge around the white. Fasten on the lower part of the face, whip stitching around the bottom; stuff and finish sewing around the top. The mouth can be improved by a running stitch of either black or white thread across the middle of the lips.

For the tail, cut a 1" strip, taper to the end of the cuff along the length of the front of the sock; seam and stuff. For the ears, cut two semi-circles from the remaining brown part of the sole of the sock. For the eyes, simply sew on eyes made from buttons or felt. For very young children, avoid using buttons and instead embroider with black thread (see diagram on next page).

Training Tip: It is good to have a finished monkey for a pattern. Some *persons* may be able to stitch and cut to make the body and other parts of the monkey. If not, these steps can be done before the activity begins. Many *persons* will be able to stuff the largest part, the body, and others can stuff the smaller parts. Plan to have extra help to make the activity fun. Many web sites have additional information, pictures, and assembly directions and tips.

The (Best) Friends Way

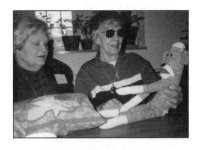

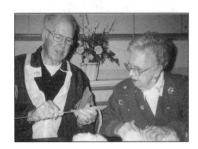

Life Story: Discuss whether a *person's* mother or father made toys by hand. What were they? Ask participants if they had a stuffed toy or teddy bear as a child? Did the family work together on projects? Did anyone work in a store that sold toys? Did someone have a German teddy bear?

Exercise: Walk to garage sales and look for "vintage" sock monkeys.

Humor: Joke about the pros and cons of having a pet monkey.

Early Dementia: Involve the *person* in the shopping process for the supplies. Ask the *person* to work with you to lead the project for others.

Late Dementia: *Persons* can enjoy holding the soft, stuffed monkey.

Sensory: The fabric of the socks is fun to handle, and the finished monkey is comforting to touch.

Spirituality: Finished monkeys can be donated to a children's charity or hospital in the spirit of giving.

Conversation: Have some fun, "Does this look like a monkey to you?" or "What does it mean to talk about monkeying around?" Reminisce, "Did you have a favorite stuffed animal when you were growing up?" Compliment, "Your toy turned out so well. Your grandson Mike is going to love that monkey!"

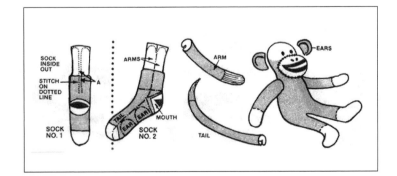

An ounce of prevention...

Divide this project into several work sessions or days. It might be overwhelming to complete in one session.

Being a Volunteer

Volunteering can fulfill a need many of us have to help others. *Persons* with dementia have the same need and have much left to give even when opportunities to help others become more and more limited.

The Basics _____

Brainstorm all of the ways for *persons* with dementia to volunteer, such as

- Befriend another individual in the day center or residential care setting (ideas include helping someone to get to a meal or an activity, walking down the hall, or holding hands to reassure or comfort someone)
- Help prepare or deliver meals to homebound individuals
- Help with office work: stamping, stuffing, and folding
- Assist in child care with a supervisor: reading, playing, listening, and loving
- Care for plants and animals
- Play the piano or lead a group in singing

The 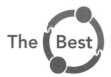 Best Friends Way _____

Life Story: Look for remaining abilities and interests to incorporate into this activity. Consider past occupations and hobbies as well as past volunteer work. Develop a group discussion on a *person's* volunteer interests such as scouting or working in a national park. Did someone volunteer for the Peace Corps, work as a docent at a museum, or volunteer at a zoo or historical society?

Exercise: Volunteering can involve much physical activity such as delivering meals, walking the dog, or playing with children.

Humor: Laugh about being a career volunteer.

Early Dementia: Continue volunteer work as long as possible with just the amount of assistance the *person* needs. Some *persons* with early dementia find satisfaction from speaking about their experience to classes and support groups.

Music: *Persons* may be able to volunteer to entertain others by singing in a choir, playing a musical instrument, dancing in a group, whistling a tune, or yodeling.

Spirituality: Being compassionate and concerned about others fulfills a spiritual need.

An ounce of prevention...

Many volunteer tasks will come to an end as the disease progresses. Activity leaders have to be able to bring closure in a very sensitive way, maybe by substituting other appropriate activities to fill the void.

Conversation: Reminisce, "You must feel really proud of all the time you spent working with those Girl Scouts." Joke, "Did you get rich volunteering?" Encourage the *person* to continue volunteering, "I need help delivering these meals. I would like for you to go with me." or "Can you help us label these newsletters?"

The Basics

- Flower blossoms
- Waxed paper, iron, crayons
- Vegetable or cheese grater
- Hole punch, string or yarn, and suction cups with hooks

Press the blossoms face down between paper towels, and place under a weight for several days. Arrange a blossom or blossoms on a sheet of waxed paper. Grate crayons into shavings and then sprinkle shavings around the blossom. Cover with a second sheet of waxed paper, and iron the two sheets together (set your iron on the lowest setting). Cut into any desired shape to include the blossom and some shavings. Punch a hole near the top edge of the sun catcher. Thread a piece of yarn or string through the hole. Hang on a windowpane using a suction-cup hook.

Variations: Tie the activity to a holiday by using a shamrock or clover for sun catchers for St. Patrick's Day or a poinsettia for Christmas.

Planning Tip: Some *persons* love to create interesting designs and will be engaged immediately in a project like this. Others like to wait until something catches their interest.

Sun Catchers

Sun catchers can be made to hang in a window, creating an effect almost like stained glass. These artistic creations brighten up the window and your mood. *Persons* with dementia can have fun making this gift for others as well as seeing sunlight peek through their artwork in a sunny window.

The 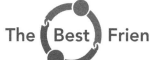 Best Friends Way

Life Story: Did anyone ever visit a cathedral in Europe and admire the wondrous stained glass? Did anyone grow up in a house with leaded glass windows?

Music: Playing relaxing background music can enhance the setting when working on this project. Alternatively, have fun and put on some bold organ music and pretend you are in a cathedral.

Old Skills: Cutting with scissors, ironing, grating, and pressing flowers are all old skills familiar to many.

Sensory: The color and the aroma of the blossoms mixed with the sounds and sights of working together can be a stimulating sensory experience.

Spirituality: Enjoy a slide show of stained-glass windows or flip through picture books.

Conversation: Encourage an opinion, "What color crayon will go well with this blossom?" Compliment your friend, "You cut your sun catcher in the shape of a heart. How creative!" Try making a deal, "I will make one of these for you if you will make one for me." Reminisce, "Did you ever have to help with the ironing when you were growing up?"

Planning an Art Show

Most of us like to see our creative art displayed. An art show evokes old social graces of entertaining. For *persons* with dementia, being able to show off their creations brings added purpose to creating the art.

The Basics

- Plan to have regular creative arts sessions and encourage participation. Think creatively and include objects other than paintings and drawings, such as poetry, sculptures, and collages.
- Encourage those who are able to sign each work of art.
- It is fun to mat the work as you go along. Some frame shops will donate framing materials.
- Decide on a time for the art show and where you will hang the works. Many places like malls, banks, and senior citizens centers welcome an exhibit. You may want to have the show at your place before it travels to give everyone an opportunity to enjoy the creations.
- Ask *persons* who would enjoy the experience to help hang the exhibit.

Planning Tip: The Alzheimer's Association's "Memories in the Making Program™" offers tips on how to create an art show (visit http://www.alzoc.org/support/memoriesprogram.htm).

The 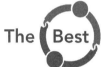 Best Friends Way

Life Story: Which *person* has loved art galleries and can tell you the famous ones he or she has visited? Who remembers art classes in school? Accept as a challenge the *person* who says that he or she cannot create anything or the families who are quick to say that their family member won't participate in any art project.

The Arts: There may be *persons* who have a good eye for displaying the works in an artistic way. Utilize their strengths.

Music: Choose some soothing background music or have a pianist or harpist perform at the art show.

Old Sayings: "A picture is worth a thousand words."

Sensory: The artwork is colorful and rich in texture to touch, and the interaction of preparing is stimulating.

Spirituality: Being able to create and have others appreciate your efforts gives a *person* a sense of accomplishment.

Conversation: Ask for opinions, "Jay, is this the right height for this picture?" Compliment, "I love this sculpture. Did you enjoy making it?" Recall a special event, "Lula, this reminds me of the photography museum in your home town of Rochester." Show appreciation, "Gladys, thanks for showing me around. You make a wonderful hostess."

An ounce of prevention...

Remember the value is in the doing. Do not leave anyone out who would enjoy seeing his or her work displayed.

The Basics —————————————

- Oranges
- Whole cloves
- Ribbon

Have a completed orange with cloves for everyone to see, smell, and touch. Stick the cloves into the orange, pointed end in first. There is no right or wrong way to arrange the cloves. Tie with a ribbon for hanging.

Discuss how the orange can be hung up in the house to make a sweet aroma during the winter months or used as a holiday ornament.

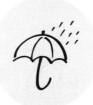

Oranges with Cloves

Can you remember the first time you saw an orange on a tree? Picked one? Tasted one? *Persons* with dementia may have a fascination with oranges; they were not as common decades ago in much of the United States as they are today. This traditional activity is easy and provides the group with a beautiful object to display in their rooms and to give to others.

The (Best) Friends Way —————————————

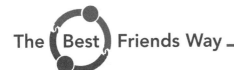

Life Story: Be familiar with the name of a family member or friend of each *person* participating and talk about making a gift for that individual, "I'll bet that your daughter, Linda, would like one of these to sweeten up the house!" or "Do you think your wife, Irene, would like a present like this?"

Exercise: This activity strengthens fine motor skills.

Early Dementia: This activity is one that a *person* can complete on his or her own.

Late Dementia: With help, most *persons* can participate. The *person* may just complete part of the orange or hold the finished product and enjoy the texture and aroma.

Sensory: Cloves have a distinctive aroma. They may remind some *persons* of spiced tea. There is also a tactile benefit of handling the cloves. A caregiver with knack will take a few moments with the *person* just to experience the sensory pleasures of an orange with cloves.

Conversation: Ask a safe question, "Where are cloves grown?" or "Did you ever put cloves in a ham to add more flavor?" Share a longing, "I wish we could pick oranges from a tree right now." Ask an opinion, "Do you like the smell of cloves?" Oranges remind many older people of the holidays of their youth. Reminisce, "Did you ever get an orange in the toe of your stocking at Christmas?"

An ounce of prevention...

If someone would rather eat the orange than do the activity, go ahead and peel an orange and enjoy it!

Baking

What does a kitchen represent to you? Preparing a special treat of food to share with another or being with friends and family in the kitchen are old traditions. With just a little help, some *persons* can experience pleasure in preparing baked goods to share with another.

The Basics

Choose an easy recipe for baking. Examples include quick breads, cookies, cupcakes, yeast bread, cakes, and pies. Have all the ingredients and utensils ready. Take special note to distribute tasks to fit the functional level of each *person*. Involve each *person* in helping you prepare the treat. Treats can be prepared to enjoy as a group and/or made for others to be a special "homemade" gift.

The 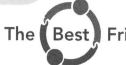 Best Friends Way

Life Story: What are the *person's* favorite baked goods? Consider regional or cultural traditions as they relate to food. Did the *person* ever work in a bakery or doughnut store? Did the *person* grow up on an apple farm, or was he or she famous for baking apple pies? Was someone a home economics major in college? Was the man the baker in the family?

The Arts: Hold a cake-decorating class or demonstration. Encourage *persons* to take their turns decorating cakes, cookies, or cupcakes.

Humor: "We should taste this before we give it away to see if it is fit to eat."

Early Dementia: *Persons* can select a recipe, do much of the baking, and help deliver the finished product.

Late Dementia: *Persons* can observe the activity, taste the finished product, and be a part of a friendly work group.

Old Sayings: "The way to a man's heart is through his stomach."

Old Skills: Rolling, beating, pouring, kneading, pounding, peeling, measuring, stirring, and reading the recipe are all old skills practiced often by many *persons*.

Sensory: Freshly baked goods fill a room with wonderful aromas and stimulate the taste buds.

Conversation: Reminisce, "Edna, did you take a pie or cake to families when a new baby was born?" Ask for information, "How did you make your yeast rolls?" Encourage sensory stimulation, "Is this too sweet?" Have fun, "Do you think we could sneak another cookie?" Discuss, "Is this loaf of bread better than store-bought?"

An ounce of prevention...

Have sugar-free baked goods for persons *on a sugar-free diet.*

The Basics

Brainstorm opportunities that *persons* might have to entertain others, such as a visit from children, the arrival of a group invited to perform, birthdays of residents and staff, or meetings and rehearsals that take place in your facility. Pick a party theme, be it an afternoon tea, "cocktail party," dessert party, or even a "tailgate party" in the parking lot or patio. Work as a group to prepare refreshments and decorate.

Choose three or four *persons* who would enjoy helping with the details of entertaining. Make invitations, perhaps on handmade paper (see page 70)

Involve *persons* who like cookie baking to help make cookies for the party. At the time of the party, invite *persons* to assume duties such as greeting guests, passing out napkins, serving refreshments, or presenting a gift.

Entertaining

Human beings are social creatures by nature. Most of us like to be with others and will go to great lengths to entertain our friends and family. *Persons* with dementia often retain their entertaining skills, making this activity a popular one.

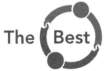

The (Best) Friends Way

Life Story: Who is very social and loves being with people? Who is the Queen or King of entertainment? Has anyone been entertained in a special place such as the White House or the Vatican? Has anyone entertained a celebrity?

The Arts: Decorate a birthday cake or wrap a gift with flair.

Humor: Laugh about company coming too soon and catching you with your hair still in curlers.

Old Sayings: "The host with the most" or "The hostess with the most-est."

Old Skills: Baking, serving refreshments, celebrating, and socializing are all old skills.

Conversation: Check with each other, "I love to have company. Don't you?" Apologize, "I'm sorry. I didn't know that you wanted to pass out the napkins." Compliment, "You work so well with children. I will know to ask you to help whenever children are invited." Ask for an opinion, "Nancy, what did you think of that banjo player? Wasn't he terrific? He liked those cookies, too."

Dog Biscuits

Many of us love animals for their ability to give unconditional love. This activity involves making tasty biscuits for our four-legged best friends. For *persons* with dementia, making dog biscuits is productive, and they can see how the product is appreciated by the dog!

The Basics

- ¾ cup hot water
- ⅓ cup margarine
- ½ cup powdered milk
- a pinch of salt
- 1 egg (beaten)
- 3 cups of whole-wheat flour

Pour the hot water over the margarine. Add the remaining ingredients and stir. Knead to form a stiff dough. Roll dough ½" thick. Cut into bone shapes, and bake at 325° for 50 minutes. Bone-shaped cookie cutters can also be purchased.

Prepare biscuits for the local animal shelter, for the dogs of friends and family members, or to give to a visiting hound! A program can also name the product "Sunshine Center Doggie Biscuits" and sell them to raise money for activities or a local charity.

The 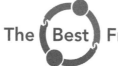 Best Friends Way

Life Story: Discover who loves dogs and who may not. Discuss favorite breeds. Some *persons* enjoy reminiscing about a favorite childhood pet. Did anyone ever enjoy attending a dog show or watching one on television like the famed Westminster Dog Show?

The Arts: Read the poem about Old Mother Hubbard aloud and write a new ending to the first verse, "Old Mother Hubbard went to the cupboard to get her poor dog a bone. When she got there, the cupboard was bare, and the poor dog had none."

Humor: Talk about how funny it is to be baking biscuits for dogs and mention that they look so good it makes everyone hungry.

Early Dementia: In addition to being very involved making the doggie bones, *persons* can also help package and deliver the finished product.

Music: Sing the song, "This Old Man" with each verse ending "with a knick knack paddy whack give a dog a bone, this old man came rolling home."

Old Sayings: "Dog tired." "Leading a dog's life." "Mean as a junkyard dog."

Sensory: The feel of the textures of the ingredients during the shaping of the biscuits is very stimulating.

Conversation: Ask an easy question, "Peggy, do you think your dog, Rover, will like one of these biscuits?" Ponder together, "Wonder what these biscuits taste like?" or "Jeremy, how did you make your biscuit look so much like a bone?" Reminisce, "Our dogs ate table scraps. Did you ever buy dog food?" Ask an opinion, "Do you approve of animals eating from the table, Elizabeth?"

CHAPTER FIVE

Games and Things to Do Together

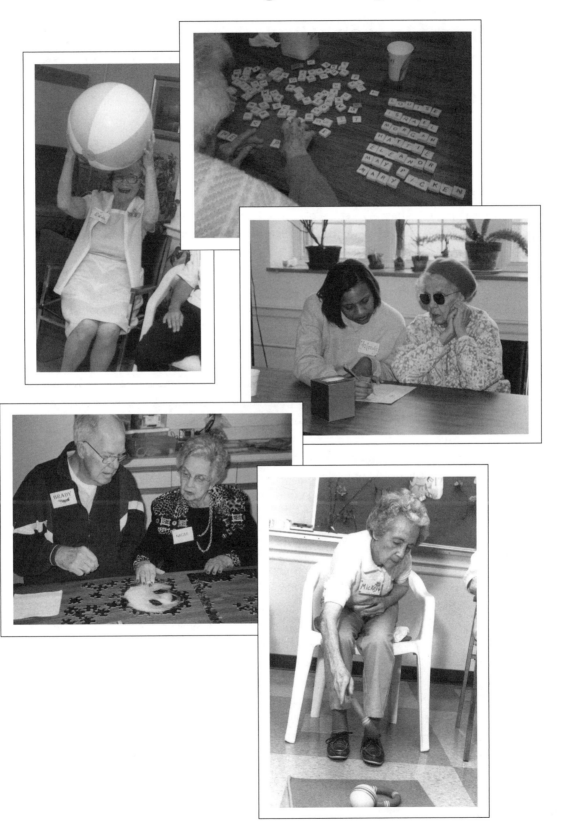

Games and
Things to Do Together

Almost all of us play games at some point in our lives, or even throughout our lives. Sometimes we play games by ourselves, such as solitaire. Other times, games are played with friends or as part of a club. Game playing has many benefits. A game can help us hone our reflexes and skills and sharpen our intellect. Games fight boredom and stress by encouraging us to become lost in a pleasurable distraction. Games can provide physical and cognitive exercise. Games can encourage teamwork and friendly competition. Success at a game can build confidence and self-esteem.

The games in this chapter have been adapted for *persons* with dementia. Specifically, a number of the games take advantage of the remaining skills many *persons* have, including:

- Retained long-term memories—Long-term memories often remain intact well into a *person's* course of dementia. Even a *person* who is quite forgetful often remembers and enjoys discussing the meaning of old sayings such as "You can lead a horse to water but… (you can't make it drink)."

- Retained physical skills—Some games in this chapter involve physical skills that remain for many *persons* with dementia, including good hand–eye coordination. *Bowling* and *Pitching and Catching* (see pages 109 and 111) are two examples that seem particularly beneficial for *persons* with dementia.

- Remaining conversational skills—A *person* may not recognize a picture of a famous person (e.g., Winston Churchill) but might still enjoy discussing the man's appearance, his hat, his frown, his wardrobe, or even the cigar he's smoking in the photograph. Once the *person* is cued that it is Winston Churchill, a conversation can ensue about the important World War II hero.

- Familiar vocabulary—*Persons* often are able to continue spelling words or playing word games. These games seem to rely on deeply learned language skills, rote memories that remain, particularly with some cueing. Thus a *person* may enjoy spelling his or her name with Scrabble tiles or responding to a word game written on a bulletin board or flip chart.

One principle of Best Friends activities is that staff and family members should enjoy the activity as much as the *person*. Caregivers with knack will take a break from their day to play and to have fun. The joyful mood that follows instills the *person* with a sense of normalcy and comforting feelings that all is well. Playing even a short but fun game can also relax the caregiver, reminding him or her of the simple joys in life that are sometimes elusive.

The chapter ends with two activities that are not traditional games but rather are things to do together—dancing and group exercises. These activities provide good physical exercise and a sense of togetherness. Do these activities before or after a game to keep the *person* (and friends, family, and caregivers) cognitively and physically active.

CHAPTER FIVE ACTIVITIES

The Basics

- Scrabble tiles, magnetic letters, or letters made out of sturdy cardboard (1" by 1" is a good size). Letter tiles can also be made using the same techniques from Clay Pinch Pots (see page 65).

Start with three or four *persons* at a table sharing a pot of assorted letters. Encourage *persons* to improvise and spell words that come to mind. Alternatively, guide group members in the spelling of their names, names of family members, or places of birth. Some will enjoy sorting letters such as gathering all the As or Bs together.

Variation: Give each *person* in the group some letters. After choosing a word such as "summer," ask Mary if she has the first letter of "summer." If Mary has an *S*, it is placed to begin the word. If not, the leader moves to the next *person*. The leader continues around the group asking for letters until the word is spelled. The leader can provide *persons* with extra letters to replenish their supply as the game progresses.

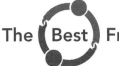

The Best Friends Way

Life Story: Working with letters around themes can help a *person* recall many happy moments such as places of birth, names of brothers and sisters, childhood games, schools attended, awards, and type of work. You will be surprised what you learn from the *person* as one memory triggers another.

Early Dementia: Ask a *person* who you know to be a good speller to help spell some difficult words.

Old Saying: "As simple as A, B, C."

Old Skills: Many *persons* pride themselves on possessing this old skill of spelling.

Spirituality: Exploring one's life helps a *person* be in touch with his or her identity, fulfilling a deep spiritual need to be known.

Conversation: Ask for help, "How do you spell your brother's name, Josiah?" Compliment often, "You are such a good speller. You must have won spelling bees at your school." Reminisce, "Ida, what was it like to have 12 children in your family?" or "Florence, you were born in Tallahassee, Florida. Can you help me spell that?"

Working with Letters

Interest in letters of the alphabet goes back to childhood when we first began to learn our ABCs. Playing games built around the use and manipulation of letters can afford many *persons* with dementia a chance to practice old skills.

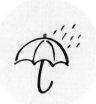

An ounce of prevention...

Keep the atmosphere light and focus on the enjoyment of creating words together. Persons can become agitated if they think they are being tested. . . Supervise so that persons don't mistake the tiles for candy.

Fun with Words

The fascination with words begins for many of us when we first learn to read. It can be surprisingly easy for *persons* with dementia to participate in word recall; it is often familiar, automatic, and implicit. This activity involves naming words to match each letter of the alphabet.

The Basics

- A list of words that could include flowers, animals, birds, proper names, gifts for different occasions, articles found in the house, occupations, or other categories
- Flip chart and markers

Begin by putting a big letter *A* on a sheet of paper or flip chart. Ask the group if they can think of a word that begins with *A* in various categories such as birds or flowers. Continue through the alphabet (e.g., *B* is for bing cherry, banana). You can work individually, in small groups of three or four, or in a larger group using a flip chart or chalkboard.

Variations: Recall all the words or phrases beginning with a color, such as the color blue: blue moon, Blue Ridge mountains, blue Monday, and Blue Danube. Or choose a single word such as *bell*, and brainstorm the many different kinds, such as wedding, ship, Liberty, school, church, and dinner.

The 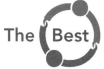 Best Friends Way

Life Story: Look for ways to connect a word in an individualized way to the *person*. If the letter is *S* and someone offers the word *salmon* and you know that Walter liked salmon fishing off the coast of Oregon in his youth, comment on that to the group.

Humor: If no one can think of an animal for a certain letter, make up a funny one, such as "Quick-as-a-wink squirrel" for the letter *Q*.

Early Dementia: Vocabulary and language skills are more intact, making this activity a successful one for many *persons*.

Spirituality: Debate the meaning of, "He is as good as his word."

Conversation: Encourage a response by saying, "Mark, I am thinking with you. How do you like the word kangaroo for the letter *K*?" Ask for information, "Is there a flower called lavender?" Give compliments, "You are very imaginative—zebra is a great animal for the letter *Z*." Rescue a *person* who has mismatched the name and the letter, "Let's save that animal, moose, for the letter *M*."

An ounce of prevention...

Persons can get upset if they feel rushed or give a wrong answer. Be prepared to step in and make any answer fit somewhere.

The Basics _____

Collect old sayings. Examples include "All that glitters is not gold" or "Birds of a feather flock together." Choose an old saying, and tell the group the first half. Ask them to complete the old saying (see the list of animal sayings on the following page for ideas).

After completing an old saying, discuss and debate its meaning. Many individuals in the group will be able to come up with a basic definition. One entertaining byproduct of this activity is that younger staff will learn phrases and old sayings they have never heard before. Younger individuals, in turn, can teach older *persons* contemporary lingo!

Variations: Engage in the activity with words that go together, such as "bread and butter," "thick and thin," or "tall, dark, and handsome." Select a "Saying of the Week" from a calendar or a book of quotations—for example, "The best thing about the future is that it comes one day at a time" (Abraham Lincoln). Display the saying in a prominent place and refer to it as often as appropriate.

Old Sayings

Knowing and using old sayings in everyday language is a part of the tradition of many older people. Because these sayings are so well-known, *persons* with dementia often can complete them better than those who are much younger.

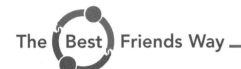

The (Best) Friends Way _____

Life Story: Use the *person's* life story to talk about some of the sayings. Some *persons* may have been reminded as teenagers that "Pretty is as pretty does" or taught their children at a young age "A penny saved is a penny earned."

Humor: Laugh and talk about the "early bird getting the worm" and wonder why anyone would want the worm.

Early Dementia: Some *persons* can lead the activity by reading the first part of an old saying for others to complete.

Late Dementia: *Persons* can sometimes still complete the phrase even after speech is quite diminished.

Conversation: Compliment, "You know all of these sayings. You've been practicing." Ask an opinion, "Is it true that 'Early to bed and early to rise makes a man healthy, wealthy, and wise'?" Provide an opportunity to teach, "Would you teach Steve that old saying… something about a 'stitch in time'?"

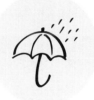

An ounce of prevention…

Some persons *can become easily frustrated if others give all of the answers. Be sure to provide an opportunity for all to participate.*

Continued on next page.

Continued from previous page.

Birds of a feather flock together

A bird in the hand is worth two in the bush

Curiosity killed the cat

Dog days of summer

You can lead a horse to water, but you can't make him drink

The early bird gets the worm

Don't look a gift horse in the mouth

Pig in a poke

Butterflies in the stomach

Bats in the belfry

Snake eyes

Whale of a good time

More fun than a barrel of monkeys

Raining cats and dogs

Kill two birds with one stone

Like a chicken with its head cut off

The best-laid plans of mice and men

The straw that broke the camel's back

Don't count your chickens before they hatch

Get your ducks in a row

Just like a pup chasing its tail

Pigging out

What's good for the goose is good for the gander

Loose as a goose

A leopard can't change its spots

Taking the bull by the horns

The cat's meow

The Basics

- Flip chart
- Colorful markers

Ask permission to print a *person's* preferred name in large-print letters vertically on a flip chart. Ask the group to think of a word that describes and compliments the *person* using each letter. For example, the name Sam can be Sensational, Sentimental, and Sassy; Appealing, Active, and Affirming; and Macho, Magnificent, and Muscular! Continue in this way until each *person* has had his or her name addressed.

Before beginning the game, brainstorm various affirming adjectives to fill in the blanks when the discussion stalls (e.g., your A list could include Appealing, Adorable, Affable, Amiable, Awesome).

Variation: Write the affirming adjectives on a card for the *person* to take home or share with others.

Training Tip: This game can be played at staff meetings to boost morale while teaching staff members how to conduct the activity.

Affirming Adjectives

Having our friends acknowledge our strengths can be affirming. *Persons* with dementia often feel that they are worthless or have diminished self-esteem because they cannot remember their many remaining abilities. This game, describing *persons* in a complimentary way, becomes very meaningful.

The (Best) Friends Way

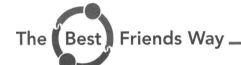

Life Story: Match elements of the *person's* life story to the activity. From the above example, the letter *S* could stand for Son of Mark and Louise, the letter *A* could stand for Architect, and *M* could stand for Married to Samantha. Strive for authenticity. If you say "best husband in the world" to someone who had a troubled marital life, it might be something the *person* will refute.

Humor: Think of humorous adjectives when you are describing a person, such as "funny," "witty," or "comical."

Spirituality: Positive descriptive words, such as "faithful church member," "kind," "loving," and "compassionate" can help a person feel appreciated.

Conversation: Encourage the group, "Maggie's name begins with the letter *M*. Let's think of a word beginning with *M* that describes Maggie." If there are no responses ask, "Do you think Maggie is Musical?" Use this opportunity to give many compliments, "What a beautiful name!" or "Your name just suits you." or "What fun to be named for your Uncle Sergio." Ask permission, "Lawrence, is it all right if I print your name on this paper? We want to say some nice things about you."

An ounce of prevention...

Be prepared if someone gives a less-than-complimentary descriptive word. Joke about the person being a "big tease" and move on.

This Is Your Life

This activity, in which the group takes time to celebrate a *person's* life, is modeled after the television program, *This Is Your Life*. This game is meaningful to *persons* with dementia because it reminds them of their life achievements and how they have touched others. This game also helps everyone in the room get to know one another in a pleasurable and interesting way.

The Basics

Gather significant information about a *person*, including props if possible, such as a special award, a quilt made by the *person*, or a picture of a *person's* rowing team in college.

Have one or two people in the group give some highlights from the *person's* life story, offer testimonials, and in general celebrate the *person's* life. If appropriate, have the *person* sit up front to receive the kind words and enjoy the props.

Finish up with a festive cake or a toast made with sparkling cider. This is a wonderful activity to celebrate a person's birthday.

Variations: Write one-sentence trivia questions about each *person* in the group and let everyone guess who it is. Examples include: "This *person* always wears blue. Who is it?" or "This *person* was born in Chile. Who is it?" A game of "This Is His or Her Life" can be played by describing a famous person and then asking the group to guess who it is.

The 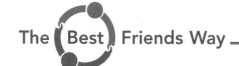 Friends Way

Life Story: This game depends on finding out as much as you can about the *person's* life. Once cued to a past success (Teacher of the Year Award or publication of an award-winning volume of poetry), *persons* often will have something to say about their life.

The Arts: Encourage participants to draw pictures or write poems about the *person* to celebrate this special occasion.

Music: Sing the *person's* favorite song.

Sensory: Pass around the props related to the *person's* life for everyone in the group to see.

Spirituality: Life review ties a *person* into his or her identity.

Conversation: Use humor, "Did you really hide your uncle's clothes while he was swimming in his birthday suit?" Give lots of compliments, "Malcolm, look at this picture of you. You have always been a good lookin' something." Ask an opinion, "Would you encourage someone today to become a car salesman?" Reminisce, "Grace, it says here that you walked 2 miles to school every day. Is that true?"

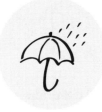

An ounce of prevention...

Sometimes persons will deny a fact about their life. Just move on when this happens— never argue!

The Basics _____

- Table games such as checkers, cards, tic-tac-toe, or puzzles (crossword, jigsaw, hidden words).

Some *persons* can work alone at solitaire or crossword and jigsaw puzzles, but most games require a teammate. Recruit staff members or volunteers to take a short break from their day and take part in the activity. The goal of these games is to help *persons* have fun and experience a measure of success.

Planning Tip: Be sensitive to the functional level of each person when choosing puzzles. Jigsaw puzzles with adult themes and a limited number of pieces usually work best.

Table Games

This activity involves playing familiar table games such as checkers, tic-tac-toe, cards, and puzzles. These games are very popular because they use old skills of *persons* with dementia, developed long ago and often still intact. This activity is a great example of how the Best Friends approach can turn something ordinary into something extraordinary.

The (Best) Friends Way _____

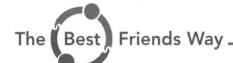

Life Story: There is no better time to talk about one's life story than when spending time together playing a game. You may find that a *person* is particularly good at playing a certain game. He or she may have won prizes or competitions. Did someone play bridge or poker? Did he or she always do the daily crossword puzzle or word jumble?

The Arts: You may want to create your own puzzles (crossword and jigsaw) or tic-tac-toe board and pieces.

Early Dementia: The *person* may be able to take part in regular games at a park or senior center, particularly if a friend provides some support.

Late Dementia: If the *person* has enjoyed card games, he or she may now enjoy sorting through the cards or even just handling them.

Old Skills: Game playing, such as checkers, involves skills that have been fine tuned through the years by many *persons*.

Sensory: The shuffling of cards, the colors of the checker board, and the feel of the game pieces all provide sensory stimulation.

Conversation: Reminisce, "Ben, did you play jacks when you were growing up?" or "What kind of games did you play in the long winter evenings when you were a boy?" Compliment, "You play Scrabble like a pro. How can you spot those words so fast?" and "You told me that you have always loved to work crossword puzzles and it shows!" Tease, "Have mercy on me. Aren't you going to let me win at least one game?" Invite the *person* to offer an opinion, "Does this puzzle piece fit in here?"

An ounce of prevention...

Be understanding with the person when he or she plays by different rules.

Lotto

An adaptation of Bingo, called Lotto, can be effective with *persons* with dementia. This activity can accommodate up to eight players; adapt as needed depending on the size of the group.

The Basics

- 50 5" by 7" index cards
- Six pictures which can be obtained from the Internet or from magazines or drawings. Good subjects include animals, birds, cars, or tools. Make sure the images have good definition and are clearly recognizable. Use a color printer or copier to make five copies of each picture, sized to fit on 5" by 8" index cards. Paste on the index cards. Keep one copy of each game card for the leader's extra set.

Shuffle the deck of cards and give each *person* five cards, making sure that no one gets two of the same kind. Begin the game with all of the picture cards face up. Call out a certain picture from your leader's set. If anyone has that particular card, he or she should turn it over. The first person to turn all of his or her cards over wins. Keep playing until everyone has won.

Planning Tip: Simple prizes like chocolates add to the fun.

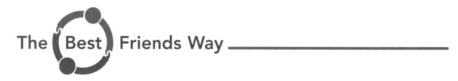

The (Best) Friends Way

Life Story: Mine the life stories of the group for ways to connect the Lotto pictures with experiences that are still meaningful to *persons*. One *person* may have a special cat, another may love cars, and another may have been handy with tools.

Early Dementia: Involve *persons* in selecting, copying, and pasting the pictures onto cards ahead of time. They can also help others during the game.

Late Dementia: A person may enjoy shuffling through the cards.

Sensory: Draw participants' attention to the colorful pictures; conversation about the colors can be very stimulating.

Conversation: Connect conversation to the life story, "Mike, you have the picture of the hammer. I know that you built the fence around your house all by yourself. You must have driven in lots of nails." Others may recall farm animals, "Here's a cow, a big Black Angus cow like Hobert's out on the farm." Reminisce, "Did you ever work on cars?" Encourage *persons* to express an opinion, "You are right. That doesn't look too much like an owl." If someone turns a picture over incorrectly, you may add, "That does look a lot like a rabbit."

The Basics

- Pictures of six to eight famous people who can be easily identified. (Oversized "coffee-table" books are often full of photographs—you can often find them discounted or on "remainder" shelves at bookstores. A color printer can also print vivid pictures from the Internet. Activity supply companies also sell sets of photographs to use in activities.)

Speculate about the lives of the people in the pictures. For example, "Does this look like someone who works with his hands?" or "Do you think she likes to shop?" Provide each *person* or team with one picture at a time to identify. Give time for each *person* or team to study the picture. Ask the group, "Who is it?"

Variation: Try "What Is It?" using photographs of famous buildings or animals. Also try "Where Is It?" using scenes from around the world.

Who Is It?

Trying to identify photographs of famous people is fun. *Persons* with dementia can be very adept at identifying pictures and can feel a sense of accomplishment in this activity.

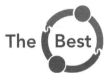

The (Best) Friends Way

Life Story: There may be *persons* who have known famous people or met some celebrity. Consider obtaining photographs of a *person's* hero or heroes or even a favorite movie star or musician. They may enjoy meaningful photographs from their own histories (e.g., photographs of Winston Churchill or Dwight Eisenhower that evoke memories of World War II).

Humor: You can laugh at the fox fur around the lady's neck in the picture or at fashions that are amusing today, such as 1960s brightly colored clothes.

Early Dementia: Many *persons* are able to help plan programs and could be a part of a work session to choose pictures of famous people to use.

Conversation: Connect with the *person's* life story, "Is it true that your father worked for Jimmy Carter?" Reminisce, "Did your Uncle Eddie really work in Hollywood in the early years?" Or "Did you ever have your portrait taken by a photographer? Was it hard sitting still for so long?" Compliment often, "I'm thinking that you must have been a good student. You have all the answers." Ask for advice, "Do you think I should grow a beard like the man in this picture?"

Charades

The well-known game of charades is adapted to be quite successful in this activity. *Persons* with dementia can respond to situations that take place in the present; they are surprisingly adept at figuring out what is being acted out without a lot of explanation.

The Basics

Develop a list of experiences that can be easily acted out by staff or by selected *persons* with dementia. A list might include fishing, jumping rope, playing a game of jacks, sweeping, eating an ice cream cone, putting on makeup, and driving a truck.

The leader acts out scenarios and may ask certain *persons* to help her or him. As the experience is demonstrated, the group is asked to guess what they see being acted out. Spend time talking about each presentation.

Variations: Look at pictures and try to guess what is happening in them.

The 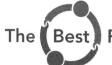 Best Friends Way

Life Story: You can use each *person's* life story to design familiar activities to act out. Act out a baseball scene for a fan of the New York Yankees or act out being a phone operator on a switchboard if someone in the group once had that job at a hotel. Also, there may be some actresses and actors in the group eager to demonstrate their talents.

Humor: Create a party atmosphere for the game, and laugh at the antics of the performers.

Early Dementia: Many *persons* will enjoy acting out one of the scenarios, such as skiing, playing hopscotch, or directing traffic.

Late Dementia: Many *persons* will be content to be a part of the fun group and watch the interaction.

Old Sayings: "Actions speak louder than words."

Sensory: Charades stimulate the visual imagination.

Conversation: Be sensitive when a *person* gives the wrong answer, "That's close." or "That's a good guess. What else could it be?" Laugh with the group, "I never thought we could have this much fun. Did you?" Reminisce about childhood games, work-related activities, and school days, "You must have played 'Ring around the Rosie' when you were a child." "I can tell that you have ridden a horse before" or "You are a natural-born actor" are great compliments.

An ounce of prevention...

Encourage persons to participate, but respect a person's desire not to take the stage.

The Basics _____

- Indoor bowling set (larger sets seem to work best)
- An adequate hallway or "alley" for rolling the bowling ball

The Process: A small group of three or four *persons* can take turns bowling, and a larger gallery can watch and cheer the bowlers, participating when they are ready. Demonstrating the game first provides a cue to the *person* as to the nature of the game.

Variation: The game can be taken outside and enjoyed as lawn bowling or "bowling on the green."

Bowling

Bowling has been a popular pastime for decades, and many individuals have competed in bowling leagues as children or adults. This is an easy skill for *persons* with dementia who find it entertaining.

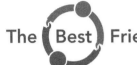

The (Best) Friends Way _____

Life Story: What qualities about each *person* can you mention while he or she is bowling—determination, fun, sense of humor, or patience? Does anyone bowl on a team or has anyone bowled a perfect 300 game? Is the person of Italian American heritage who might have enjoyed playing bocci ball? Is someone from New Zealand where he or she played lawn bowling?

Exercise: Bowling is great to get *persons* moving. It strengthens the upper body even if the person is bowling from a chair.

Early Dementia: Encourage the person to go out to bowl with family and friends or a league if that has been his or her interest.

Old Sayings: "He or she is a good sport." "Gutterball."

Sensory: The feel of the bowling ball and the laughter and fun conversation make for a sensory-filled time together.

Conversation: This is a good time to reminisce, "Trish, did you ever bowl when you were a little girl?" or "Did you have a bowling alley in your home town of Corning, Iowa?" "Compliment often, "You really have a strong arm" or "You have a good eye." Try teasing, "You are making me work very hard. You are too good at knocking down all those pins!" Ask for opinions, "Do I have the pins set up correctly? Should they be farther apart?" Encourage everyone to take turns, "Lift this ball. Isn't it heavy? Try rolling it right down this way."

An ounce of prevention...

If a person's balance is impaired, steady him or her during bowling or let him or her roll the ball from a sitting position.

Horseshoes

Tossing horseshoes is a tradition in rural America and has been played by countless people in summer camps or on family holidays. Tossing horseshoes is a satisfying activity for *persons* with dementia because it is a familiar movement.

The Basics

- An indoor horseshoe game (one with light plastic horseshoes and a stake that is on a stand)
- Arrange chairs in a circle so everyone can enjoy seeing each *person* as he or she takes a turn tossing the horseshoes.

Variations: Use colorful rings to toss at the horseshoe stake. A 2" by 2" piece of carpet can also be used as the target.

A 1-gallon plastic container makes a good target for tossing beanbags. Use three 1-gallon containers and challenge the group to get one beanbag in each container.

The 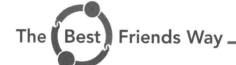 Best Friends Way

Life Story: For each *person's* turn, begin by calling the *person* by name. Use the life story to give a fact about each *person's* life. It may be where the *person* was born or some special event in the *person's* life, such as being the father of twin boys or a more recent happening such as a new hairstyle. "Mr. Somberg, it's your turn to throw the horseshoe. [To the group] Mr. Somberg owned the best hardware store in Milwaukee."

Exercise: Tossing horseshoes can be done from either a standing or a sitting position and is excellent exercise for the upper body.

Early Dementia: Many *persons* enjoy being in charge of moving the targets from one *person* to the next.

Late Dementia: Move the target very close or assist *persons* in tossing.

Old Sayings: "Ringer." "Leaner."

Sensory: Bring in a real horseshoe to touch and discuss.

Conversation: Reminisce about playing horseshoes, "Did just the men play horseshoes?" or "Did they use real horseshoes?" Ask advice, "You are so good at making a ringer. I need your advice. Am I holding these rings the right way?" Use humor whenever possible, "Look where those rings landed. You don't know your own strength! We are all so good. We'll have to take our show on the road." Compliments are always in vogue, "Congratulations, you just hit the bull's eye again." Discuss trivia, "Is there a right way and a wrong way to hang a horseshoe on the wall for good luck?" (Up, so the luck won't run out.)

The Basics

- A small basketball or other soft ball
- A basketball hoop, small trash can, basket, or other container to be a "goal" for the ball toss

Arrange chairs in a circle so everyone can enjoy games of throwing or catching. Take turns to shoot for the goal or play toss with one another. This game also works well one-to-one.

Variations: Take a small group to a softball game to enjoy watching or watch a Frisbee toss at a park. Velcro darts and a dartboard can be used indoors.

The 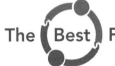 Best Friends Way

Life Story: Most everyone has some connection to either baseball or basketball. Softball was a popular Sunday afternoon diversion, and many families attended the games. Did someone collect baseball cards as a child? Does someone have a grandchild active in Little League? Who had a basketball hoop in his or her backyard?

Exercise: This is excellent exercise, especially if *persons* are able to be more active for participation, such as throwing a Frisbee, shooting basketball hoops, or playing catch out of doors.

Humor: "You hit that one out of the ballpark."

Early Dementia: Continue playing on a softball team or attending local sports events.

Music: Sing the song, "Take Me Out to the Ballgame."

Old Sayings: "Hitting the bull's eye." "Seventh-inning stretch."

Old Skills: *Persons* with dementia often retain the skills of throwing and catching, particularly when given cueing and encouragement.

Conversation: Invite, "Let's toss the ball back and forth for awhile." Reminisce, "What kind of uniforms did the basketball players wear when you were in high school? Did you ever hit a home run in baseball?" Ask opinions, "Do you like the basketball hoop right here? Is this good for you?" Compliment, "You made that basket like an old pro." Utilize some knack to get a reluctant *person* to play ball, "Bill, I have a big game Sunday. Would you help me practice?"

Batting a Balloon

This simple activity involving a balloon is surprisingly fun and can be started on the spot by a caregiver with a balloon in his or her pocket and five or six puffs of air! The balloon costs 5 cents, but the value to *persons* with dementia can be immeasurable.

The Basics

Arrange chairs in a circle and invite the group to sit. Choose a large colorful balloon and blow it up. Begin batting the balloon. Have a staff member in the middle of the circle to steer the balloon to everyone and keep the balloon "in play." Call each *person* by name as the balloon comes to them and add a piece of biographical information each time, "Now the balloon is with John. John loves strong coffee and doughnuts!"

Variation: This is also a simple one-to-one activity. Velcro balls and paddles can be used with the same batting motion as with batting a balloon. Other active games include kicking a beach ball and indoor golf putting. Order a balloon bouquet for a special birthday or anniversary

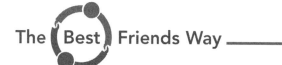

The (Best) Friends Way

Life Story: What memories do balloons hold for *persons*? Birthdays, circuses, county fairs, carnivals? Did any *person* ever ride in a hot-air balloon or see a blimp?

Exercise: Batting a balloon stretches the chest, upper arms, and even the legs as individuals catch a missed balloon with their hands or feet.

Late Dementia: Hold your hands over the hands of the *person* to help catch the balloon.

Music: Bat the balloon to the rhythm of music.

Sensory: Balloons come in an array of colors and have a distinctive feel; sometimes they make a squeaky noise when caught.

Conversation: Reminisce by saying, "Did you ever lose your balloon and watch as it floated into the sky?" "Did you ever ride in a hot-air balloon?" Compliment, "You've got a good batting arm. Did you play baseball?" Encourage, "That balloon is an escape artist. Try again." Think of something humorous, "You almost fell out of your chair but you made that hit!" Ask an opinion, "Do you like the red balloon or the yellow balloon best?"

An ounce of prevention...

Some persons may become fearful when the balloon is batted toward them. Use caution and common sense.

The Basics _____

- Some strange gadgets or odds and ends, such as a strawberry huller, a wooden massager, a shoe buttoner, a candle snuffer, a buckeye, a car oil changer, a dinosaur gizzard stone, a corn-on-the-cob butterer.

Inspiration can be found at garage sales or dollar stores! The possibilities are endless! Ask staff and family to contribute to your collection of odd items. Many of the items may be antique gadgets and tools that some *persons* in your group recognize.

Pass the items around one at a time. Have group members guess what each object is. If someone knows, encourage him or her to share with the group and demonstrate its usage. If no one knows, see if the group can make something up!

Variation: Place familiar articles in a paper bag and let *persons* guess what they are by reaching into the bag and examining them without looking in the bag.

Have you ever found a gadget at home and thought, "What is this?" This game does just that by showing strange objects and opening the group's imagination to what it could possibly be. *Persons* with dementia enjoy this game because there is no right or wrong answer to the question of "What is it?"

The 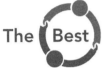 Best Friends Way _____

Life Story: Try to find items that will relate to the life stories of your group participants, such as farm tools for the farmer, kitchen tools for the *person* who likes to cook, knickknacks for the collector.

The Arts: Arrange an exhibit of the unusual objects you have collected and continue the discussion of "What is it?"

Humor: Make up funny names such as "flea catcher" or "thingamabob" for items that you can't figure out.

Old Sayings: "One man's trash is another man's treasure!"

Sensory: Look at, listen to, and feel the items to try to figure out what they are used for.

Conversation: The following general questions work well: "What in the world is this?"; "What was this used for?"; "Has anyone ever owned or used one of these?"; "Where do you find something like this?" Encourage, "I promise there is nothing in the bag that will hurt you." Compliment someone, "You're good—I would have never figured that out!" Encourage a *person* to teach the group, "Martin, we would all like to learn how to use that one. Would you show us how it works?"

Let's Dance

Many people have fond memories of dancing, whether it is the jitterbug, the waltz, free-form at a rock-and-roll concert, or a slow dance with a date. *Persons* with dementia who have enjoyed dancing may appreciate the joy and intimacy that comes from partaking in this activity.

The Basics

- Music for dancing (A piano player or musician is ideal, but taped music will suffice.)
- Staff or volunteers to assist as partners

Create a fun atmosphere for the dance and utilize staff volunteers as dance partners. Try to involve everyone, taking care to not ignore *persons* on the sidelines.

The  Best Friends Way

Life Story: Some *persons* may be excellent dancers and enjoy different kinds of dances. Learn about a *person's* favorite type of music for dancing. Did anyone take dancing lessons—tap, ballet, or ballroom, perhaps from the famed Arthur Murray schools? Others may have never had an opportunity to dance, or thought they were not good dancers.

Exercise: Movement to music is one of the best exercises.

Humor: Talk about having "two left feet." Laugh about dancing just like Fred Astaire and Ginger Rogers.

Early Dementia: Encourage a *person* who loves dancing to continue with a partner or in a dance group.

Late Dementia: Some *persons* enjoy swinging and swaying to the music from their chair or wheelchair with help from a partner.

Old Skill: Dancing is an old skill that is easily renewed.

Sensory: Listening to music, feeling the warm touch of a dance partner, and tapping your toes to the rhythm of the music tickles the senses.

Conversation: Share your memories, "Helen, did you have school dances when you were growing up?" Ask for help, "Can you teach me how to waltz?" Compliment, "Mona, you are so graceful as you dance around the room. You are a wonderful dancer!" Share your concern, "I have trouble following. I am always stepping on my partner's toes. I think I need dancing lessons." Ask for an opinion, "Natasha, do you like to dance to fast or slow music?"

An ounce of prevention...

Some persons' religious practices prohibit dancing. Be respectful of differences.

114

The Basics ⎯⎯⎯⎯⎯⎯⎯⎯⎯⎯⎯

Arrange chairs in a circle, allowing plenty of room for *persons* to stretch. Invite *persons* to join the group. If the word *exercise* has a negative connotation, use knack and call it a "movement class." It is best to let *persons* sit while exercising. More active *persons* can exercise by walking in addition to the sitting exercises.

The leader sets the tone for a successful time together. It is important to talk about the value of exercise and at the same time exude enthusiasm for a fun time together. Encourage and model the various exercises.

Planning Tip: This can be a time of socialization by sharing stories, laughing, and talking together.

The Best Friends Way ⎯⎯⎯⎯⎯⎯⎯⎯

Life Story: Call *persons* by name as you go through the routines. Think about each *person's* life story. What do you know about each *person* that is related to exercise? Was a *person* in the army? Can he or she lead the marching? Who is a walker, a runner? Who did physical labor using their strength to make a living? Who can demonstrate playing the piano to exercise your hands? Who can count in a different language as you count off the strokes? Become familiar with those *persons* who like to lead a certain exercise.

Humor: Joke about having an 18" waistline after twisting and turning.

Late Dementia: *Persons* who have difficulty following directions can be helped by taking their hands and exercising together.

Music: Exercise by moving to music. Use scarves to wave to the rhythm of the music and encourage upper-arm exercises.

Old Skills: Many *persons* will recall calisthenic exercises. These movements will be familiar.

Sensory: Exercise puts *persons* in touch with their bodies and sharpens their senses.

Conversation: Encourage, "Mariah can you lift your feet up so we can all see your new cross-training shoes." Use the life story, "Mark, you are an old army man. Can you help us march?" Seek assistance, "Harry, we need your help to count to 10 in German as we stretch our arms." Give a compliment as hands are being exercised, "Good, Joe, that's exactly the way to 'play the piano.' You would make a great pianist." Asking for an opinion makes great conversation, "Is this the way to row a boat?"

An ounce of prevention...

The staff member needs to be aware of any restrictions on exercise for individuals.

115

CHAPTER SIX

Personal Care as an Activity

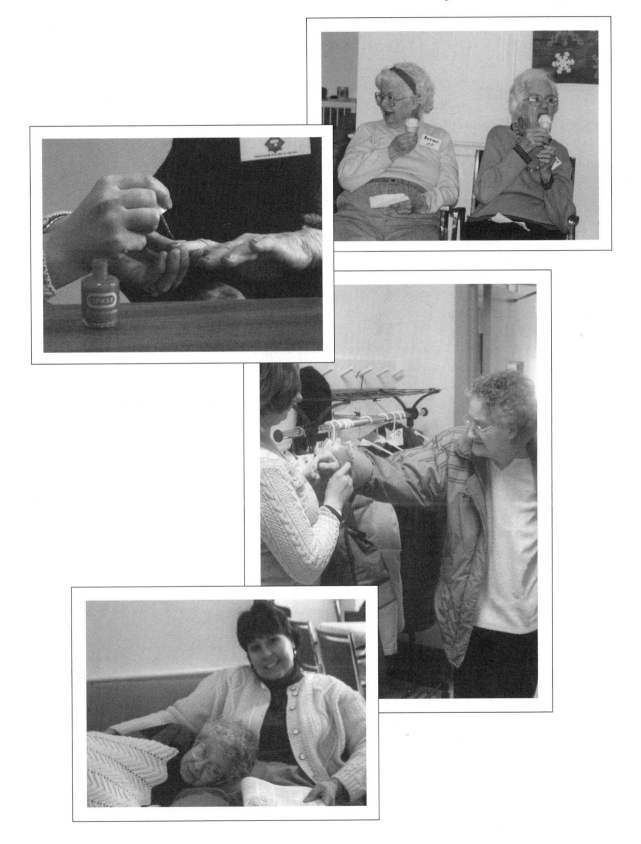

Personal Care as an Activity

Personal care, whether it is bathing, dressing, brushing teeth, shaving, or going to the bathroom, is a part of everyone's daily routine. When we are on top of these chores, we generally look and feel our best. Alzheimer's disease and other dementias gradually transform personal care from a private pursuit to one in which the *person with dementia* eventually needs assistance from a caregiver.

Maintaining personal care can be quite challenging. *Persons* with memory loss and confusion may have forgotten their past routines or may not understand the need to brush their teeth or go to the bathroom regularly. The *person* may be reluctant to let a caregiver help with such private matters. In residential care facilities and private homes alike, caregivers struggle to find a delicate balance between helping the *person* keep as much independence as possible while providing the amount of assistance that is needed.

The activities described in this chapter can help you address this situation. Personal care becomes more than tasks to be completed, baths to be given, or food to be eaten, but a time to savor the fragrance of the soap, enjoy the feeling of the warm water, taste a familiar comfort food, and reminisce about dinner activities around the old family table. Introducing gentle touch and conversation into activities such as bathing, toileting, and grooming can help ease the uncomfortable feeling of having a caregiver present during previously private activities.

The activities in this chapter encourage you to make a connection with the *person* before embarking on a personal-care task. This may only take a few minutes but will increase the odds of success dramatically. A good example is *Bathing* (see page 124). If you are helping a *person* take a bath and follow the suggestions offered in that activity, the initial 5 minutes you spend becoming friends will speed up the task. A few general principles apply when you are helping a *person with dementia* with personal care:

- Be flexible: If the person is rushed in personal care, both the caregiver and the person may become frustrated and the interaction may be poor. Make sure to allow enough time for the person to function at his or her highest level.
- Show dignity and respect: Remember that it can be difficult to have someone else present during private personal-care tasks. Take every step to make sure that you communicate respect and ensure dignity during the activity.
- Maintain routines: Honor lifelong habits regarding personal care. This includes the time of day in which a *person* is accustomed to completing the task.
- Plan ahead: Make sure to set up the personal care activity for success. Prepare the environment ahead of time by having everything you need within arm's reach.
- Step in: Use finesse to protect dignity when trying to help a *person* who has spilled food or whose sweater may be inside-out.

Many books and training programs are solely devoted to the dos and don'ts of personal care. We assume that staff will receive this basic training. Nevertheless, each activity in this chapter briefly introduces the topic and covers some of the basics of personal care and discusses how to transform the personal-care task into a meaningful activity. Invaluable conversation starters follow that will help staff begin the activity on the right foot.

If staff practice these techniques, they will develop knack and understand that quality care only becomes possible when they become less task oriented and more person *oriented*.

CHAPTER SIX ACTIVITIES

The Basics

Prepare for the meal ahead of time by planning for foods and utensils that fit the *person's* functional level. Create a café atmosphere by using smaller tables, colorful tablecloths, and flowers. Many *persons* prefer a quiet atmosphere that facilitates table talk. Consider adopting flexible serving schedules to accommodate each *person's* routines.

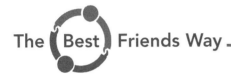

The Best Friends Way

Life Story: Know the *person's* likes and dislikes. Respect the *person's* cultural background, which may affect the types of food served and dining traditions. Was the *person* a cook or chef? Did the *person* consider her- or himself an adventuresome diner or someone who liked "meat and potatoes?" Does the *person* do better eating in a group setting or on his or her own?

Late Dementia: If a *person* needs assistance with eating, position yourself at his or her eye level, establish good eye contact, and call the *person* by name.

Music: Sometimes playing a certain song or type of music to denote each meal (e.g., classical at breakfast) helps establish a comforting routine.

Old Sayings: "A spoonful of sugar helps the medicine go down." "Too many cooks spoil the broth."

Sensory: Admire the colors on the plates, placemats, napkins, and flowers. Enjoy the smell of freshly baked bread. Discuss the taste of creamy mashed potatoes and gravy.

Spirituality: Encourage the *person* to pray before eating if that is his or her tradition, or, if appropriate, say a prayer with the *person*.

Conversation: Ask for help, "Would you lend me your recipe for lasagna?" Share a common interest, "Javier, I love Mexican food, too. Do you like it mild or really spicy?" Ask an opinion, "Do you like apple or cherry pie best?" If the person needs help, intervene with little fanfare, "Is it okay if I help you, you have a little food on your mouth?" Gently and discreetly wipe it off with a tissue or cloth.

Let's Eat

Is eating a highlight of your day? Many of us start thinking about what to have for lunch as soon as breakfast is finished. A caregiver with knack makes the most of mealtime and uses this sensory and pleasurable activity as an opportunity for meaningful interactions with *persons* with dementia.

An ounce of prevention…

Be sure to place the person *close enough to the table to allow for maximum independence and prevention of spills. During the meal remain alert to the needs of* persons *and offer assistance as needed.*

Toileting

Have you ever needed assistance with going to the bathroom, perhaps during an illness or after an injury? The *person* with dementia has a need for privacy in the bathroom, but also gradually needs more and more assistance as dementia progresses.

The Basics

Make the bathroom as inviting and home-like as possible, while employing good lighting and grab bars. Soft background music can be pleasant. Pay special attention to maintaining dignity by noting the following guidelines.

- Discreetly ask the *person* if he or she needs to go to the bathroom
- Provide as much privacy as possible
- Never scold or shame for accidents
- Never rush the *person*

Establish a routine to prevent accidents. However, if the *person* becomes incontinent, obtain a complete medical evaluation to see if it can be treated or corrected. Learn all you can about current products that can make caring for incontinence much easier (e.g., incontinence briefs, creams and lotions, clean-up products, deodorants).

The 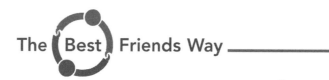 Best Friends Way

Life Story: Use familiar words for toileting (e.g., "powder your nose" for ladies, "go to the head" for an ex-Navy officer). Maintain past behaviors, patterns, and routines. Use some fact from the *person's* past to build trust while conversing with him or her in the bathroom (e.g., talk about a favorite type of music, sports team, or shared interest).

Humor: Use self-deprecating humor. Say "I seem to be all thumbs today" when helping someone zip up, or joke about having cold hands.

Late Dementia: When a *person* is wearing incontinence briefs or aids, maintain dignity by calling the *person* by his or her preferred name, empathizing with the *person's* feelings, showing patience, and respecting privacy as much as possible.

Conversation: If *persons* are reluctant to use the bathroom, ask, "Virginia, would you take a walk with me?" and then steer her toward the bathroom. Ask for some company, "Mom, I have to go to the bathroom. Come with me so we can wash up together." Ask permission, "May I help you with your slacks?" Have a light touch, "Anyone can have an accident."

An ounce of prevention...

Having an effective caregiving plan when away from home can help a person avoid accidents and makes life easier for everybody. Patronize restaurants or other shops with family-friendly, unisex bathrooms.

The Basics

Some individuals may be able to dress on their own; others will need more help. If the *person* needs assistance, lay out some ideas for clothes for the day and give as many cues as needed to help the *person* dress. You may need to hand him or her one item of clothing at a time and give cues about how to proceed. Take the time to talk to the *person* about his or her clothing. Ideally, let the *person* get dressed on his or her schedule—don't rush.

Training Tip: At a staff meeting, role play or brainstorm the various steps involved in getting dressed. Ask how long it will take for staff to get up and get dressed in the morning. This helps staff appreciate the complexity of dressing.

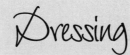

Dressing

Are you a "clotheshorse," someone who loves shopping for and wearing clothes? Many people spend a great deal of time (and money) planning their wardrobes. *Persons* with dementia are no different, and the daily activity of getting dressed can be transformed from another task to a pleasurable activity.

The 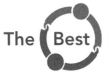 Best Friends Way

Life Story: Mine the life story to understand if the *person* sewed her own clothes. Did she have a seamstress or buy clothes off the rack? Did the *person* wear a uniform? Does the woman enjoy a fancy hat? Does the man detest wearing a necktie or enjoy dressing up? Did the *person* enjoy reading fashion magazines or spend hours at dress shops? Did the *person* enjoy going to big sales or did he or she buy something no matter what the price?

Early dementia: Let the *person* choose what he or she wants to wear, even if it doesn't conform to traditional fashion sense.

Late Dementia: Make sure the *person* has warm and comfortable clothes.

Old Sayings: "Clothes make the man." "A stitch in time saves nine." "Sunday best."

Sensory: Give a shoulder massage when helping put on a shirt or blouse if the *person* enjoys it. Give a foot massage as you put on socks.

Conversation: Ask an easy question, "That shirt has such pretty colors, is it new?" Give a compliment, "Lon, you look great in red!" Ask for advice, "How do you put a hem in?" Ask for an opinion about something you are wearing, "Do you think this matches?" Be self-deprecating, "I'm having a bad hair day, do you think I should put on a hat?" Debate, "Do you think store clerks treat you better if you go in well dressed?"

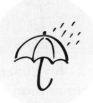

An ounce of prevention...

Clean out the closets! Eliminate clothing that is no longer worn or too complex to put on and take off easily (for example, clothes with too many buttons or zippers). This helps simplify choices.

Bathing

Do you enjoy a hot bath or an invigorating shower? Bathing is a regular chore but also a pleasurable activity for most of us. With a sensitive, creative approach, *persons* with dementia may enjoy the experience, rather than resisting a bath or shower.

The Basics

Try to maintain a home-like environment by having plush bathmats, plants, or pictures on the wall. Be sure the room is warm and free of drafts. Organize your supplies so that you don't waste time or keep a restless *person* waiting while you search for shampoo, towels, or soap. Review the bathing area—would *you* feel comfortable being bathed in this environment?

Assess the *person's* bathing needs. Not everyone needs daily bathing. Consider alternate bathing options when showers or baths are difficult. These can include bed and towel baths, soap-less baths, and other products available from medical-supply companies or from home health agencies. In residential settings, hold a case conference to explore options and ideas if staff members struggle with bathing a person.

Planning Tip: Many of the principles in this activity also relate to washing or shampooing a *person's* hair.

The (Best) Friends Way

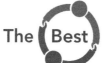

Life Story: Maintain past behaviors, patterns, and routines, such as the type of bath, the time of day, and the frequency. Did the *person* take a quick shower in the morning before rushing off to work or take a leisurely bath at the end of each evening? Use familiar phrases such as "to wash up" or "to freshen up."

Music: Play some familiar background music in the bathing room.

Old Sayings: "Clean as a whistle." "Cleanliness is next to godliness."

Sensory: Warm relaxing water; the clean smell of perfumed soap; and a fluffy, comforting towel can provide sensory pleasure. The tone of your voice when inviting a *person* to bathe can make all the difference.

Conversation: Ask an opinion, "Is the water warm enough?" Reminisce, "On the farm where you grew up, where was the bathtub?" Employ humor, "Erlene, isn't it fun to get in here and get all scrubbed up?" Reassure, "I'm right beside you. I won't let you fall." Encourage, "I can't wait to have tea and cookies as soon as your bath is all finished. Doesn't that sound good to you?"

An ounce of prevention...

Encourage staff to be empathetic; bathing can be scary (fear of falls), embarrassing (nudity), and uncomfortable (arthritis, pain, cold). Don't let your bathroom become too institutional in its appearance or a place for storage for unused equipment and supplies!

The Basics

Washing hands is very important. If the *person* is reluctant to do this, use a waterless antibacterial gel to get the *person's* hands clean. A nailbrush can be used to clean nails. Give the *person* a hand massage using lotion.

If the *person* wishes, give a full manicure by trimming, filing, and painting his or her nails.

Variation: Many of the ideas in this activity also apply to foot care.

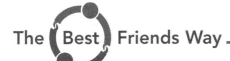

The Best Friends Way

Life Story: Talk about all the things the person's hands have done throughout the person's life, such as raising children, designing buildings, typing letters, or writing on the chalkboard. Admire someone's rings and try to learn their history (was a turquoise ring given to someone by a tribal leader or did she buy her amber ring in Africa?)

Early Dementia: Ask the person to give you a manicure!

Old Sayings: "The hand that rocks the cradle is the hand that rules the world." "Caught red-handed." "Don't bite the hand that feeds you." Talk about words that include *hand*, such as *handmade, hand-me-down, farmhand,* and *handful.*

Sensory: Enjoy the scent of the lotion. Admire the bright, sparkly colors of the nail polish and the soothing feeling of a hand massage. Enjoy the weight and sight of a decorative wristwatch or ring.

Spirituality: Holding a hand evokes feelings of love and intimacy.

Conversation: Reminisce, "Did you ever go to a salon for a manicure?" Ask an opinion, "Elna, do you like the smell of this lotion? It smells like vanilla to me, what do you think?" or "I think this pink polish will look nice with your shirt. What do you think?" Discuss what it means to have rough, callused hands versus smooth hands (e.g., how it might reflect the kind of work or lifestyle of a man or woman). Ask permission, "May I do your fingernails?"

Hand Care

Have you ever paused and looked at your hands? If someone has rough, callused hands he or she has likely worked in physical labor or other hard work. Someone with soft hands may have traveled a different career or life path. In any case, the hand is a remarkable part of being human, and hand care is a wonderful way to connect to the *person* with dementia.

An ounce of prevention...

If the person has diabetes or a nail infection, make sure to consult a physician first for proper hand (or foot) care and technique.

A Close Shave

What does shaving represent to men? It's a ritual that most men have done for nearly all of their lives. Men with dementia may still enjoy the feeling of being freshly shaved. Here is an activity that makes shaving a rich, sensory, and successful activity.

The Basics

Gather all necessary equipment before beginning: razor, shaving cream, shaving brush, towels, warm water, aftershave, and beard trimmer. Establish a daily routine. Before and during shaving, engage in intentional conversation. Afterward, apply healing face cream or aftershave lotion if the man used that product.

The 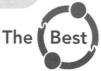 Best Friends Way

Life Story: Check to be sure that shaving is part of the *person's* cultural or religious tradition or lifestyle. Does he prefer using an electric razor? Did he ever have a mustache or a beard? Did he ever go to the barbershop for a shave?

Humor: Laugh about the "tall tales" told at the barbershop.

Early Dementia: Let the man do as much by himself as possible. Intervene for safety or the final touch up.

Music: Sing the ditty, "A shave and a haircut…two bits."

Old Sayings: "A close shave." See if you can remember any of the Burma Shave signs (Hinky Dinky, Parley Voo, Cheer Up Face, The War is Through, Burma Shave).

Old Skills: Shaving may remain an intact skill.

Sensory: The warmth of the water and towel on his face may be soothing and comforting. The smell and feel of aftershave may bring back old memories.

Conversation: Ask an open-ended question, "How do you think barbershop quartets got started?" Ask an opinion, "Did you have a favorite aftershave?" Discuss various beard types and whether he would ever grow a mustache, beard, or goatee. Reminisce, "Did your father or grandfather shave with a straight edge razor?" or "Who taught you how to shave?"

An ounce of prevention…

If he is resistant, talk with him about getting ready for the day and all of the things you will be doing. Consider trying an electric razor, even if he has never used one. Be open to new ideas—perhaps a beard would look distinguished!

The Basics

Ask a *person's* permission to brush his or her hair. Suggest that you want the *person* to look his or her best today. Using a soft, rubber-tipped brush, brush the *person's* hair gently. This is traditionally an activity for women more than men, but men may enjoy having their hair combed or brushed or being encouraged to do it themselves with some assistance. Compare two different hairbrushes and discuss the merits of each one.

Hair Brushing & Combing

Have you ever had your hair brushed or combed? It can be a very relaxing experience. *Persons* with dementia, who may have trouble doing this task on their own, may be calmed by this activity.

The 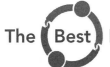 Best Friends Way

Life Story: Did the *person* have regular appointments at the beauty salon? Discuss the styles they've had over the years and what they now prefer. Look at old pictures of the *persons* in your activity or old pictures from magazines and enjoy recalling hair styles such as Afros, mullets, braids, perms with tight curls, marcelled waves, bobs, and other looks, many of which go in and out of style even today.

Humor: Joke about a military crew cut or a bad hairdo.

Late Dementia: This activity helps relax the *person* and is a good opportunity to spend quality time with the *person*.

Old Saying: "I'm having a bad hair day."

Old Skills: Hair brushing or fixing one's hair is an old skill for many. Allow them to brush their own hair or even yours. They may enjoy braiding or brushing a child's hair.

Sensory: Use a brush specially designed for scalp massage to increase tactile stimulation.

Conversation: Give a compliment, "You have such beautiful hair. What do you do to keep it so healthy?" Ask an opinion, "José, do you like my new haircut? Should I keep it long or cut it short?" Ask an easy question, "Mrs. Franklin, they used to say you should brush your hair 100 strokes every night to keep it healthy. Do you think that's true?" Ask for help, "Mom, would you brush my hair?"

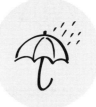

An ounce of prevention…

Ask for permission. Some persons do not like their hair to be touched or would find it painful to have their hair combed or brushed.

127

Make-Up

Are you a woman who won't go to the front doorstep for the newspaper without lipstick? Many women with dementia retain their fashion sense and want to look their best.

The Basics

Lay out the regular items the *person* uses. Help her as needed with applying her make-up. If the job becomes very difficult, gradually adapt the use of make-up to simplify her look. Lipstick is something many women enjoy and can be applied throughout the day (by the person or with assistance).

Variation: Sorting through and discussing make-up supplies can be a fun activity.

The 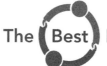 Best Friends Way

Life Story: Did she wear make-up every day or just for special occasions? What type of make-up did she wear regularly (blush, lipstick, mascara)? Was she someone who perhaps never wore much, if any, make-up? What interest does she now have in make-up, if any? Reminisce about the brand of make-up the person used or still uses (e.g., Revlon, Estée Lauder, or Mary Kay).

Early Dementia: It is easy to confuse similarly packaged make-up such as lipliner and eyebrow pencil. Supervise the *person*, but encourage independence whenever possible.

Late Dementia: Applying lipstick is often a simple, quick activity that some *persons* can do themselves.

Old Saying: "Beauty is only skin deep."

Sensory: The feel of make-up being applied can be very relaxing. Cold cream is aptly named and is usually considered very refreshing.

Conversation: Reminisce, "When did you start wearing make-up?" or "Do you remember when you bought powder loose and used a powder puff to apply it?" Have a history discussion, "Who do you think invented make-up? Who thought up wearing blue on your eyelids? Why is it called make-up anyway?" Debate, "Josephine, what are the nicest shades of lipstick?" Discuss a silly make-up name, "This lipstick is called 'Fire Engine Red.' How do you think they came up with that name?" Ask an opinion, "Do you like my new shade of lipstick? Is it too bright?" Be philosophical, "Do we wear make-up for ourselves or to look good for others?"

An ounce of prevention…

A person's cultural background, life experience, or even religion may influence their attitudes toward make-up. Be certain that you are tying the activity into the person's life story and be respectful of her values.

The Basics

Maintain a daily routine. Use a favorite toothpaste and a soft toothbrush for comfort. Encourage as much independence as possible, although many *persons* will need you to take out the toothbrush, put on the toothpaste, hand it to them, and get them started. When more help is needed, brush slowly and explain the process along the way. Brush your teeth beside the *person* to model the activity.

Dental care can become a challenge if the *person* does not understand. Break the process down into small steps and sessions. Consult a dentist for additional dental care options.

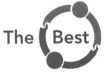

The (Best) Friends Way

Life Story: Use something from the *person's* life story as an icebreaker to build a bond of trust (talking about a favorite soap opera or hymn). Talk about how he or she might have encouraged children to brush their teeth in the past.

Early Dementia: Encourage *persons* to keep up with regular dental appointments and prompt them to brush their teeth after meals or as part of their regular routine.

Late Dementia: Be flexible. Encourage the *person*, but accept what he or she can tolerate at any one time. Mouthwash can be a way to get some extra cleansing.

Music: Playing soothing music or the *person's* favorite type of music in the bathroom can create a more pleasant atmosphere, encouraging the *person* to stay in the bathroom area longer.

Sensory: The zippy taste of mint toothpaste can be an eye opener. There is nothing like the feel of clean teeth.

Conversation: Compliment the *person* by saying "Carlos, you have such a pretty smile and pretty teeth." Help initiate the activity with knack, "Let's get ready for the day. I will brush my teeth with you." Encourage the *person*, "The dentist says we need to make sure to reach those teeth all the way in the back." Recall together getting braces for children or grandchildren.

An ounce of prevention...

Dental care often gets neglected as dementia worsens. Recognize that tooth and gum problems as well as ill-fitting dentures can cause pain, leading to agitation and combativeness.

Moving and Stretching

Our bodies are made of many moving parts that need to move and stretch to stay healthy. We can utilize personal-care activities as a friendly excuse to incorporate movement into daily routines of *persons* with dementia.

The Basics

Don't provide excessive personal care that creates dependency. This diminishes the moving and stretching that can naturally become a part of a *person's* fitness. In general, encourage each *person* to manage his or her personal care as much as possible.

When the *person* can no longer handle personal care on his or her own, be sensitive to the *person's* need to stretch and move. Use dressing as a time to give verbal prompts about stretching arms and legs. Make brushing teeth a time to shake wrists and stretch the fingers. After toileting, suggest that the *person* smooth his or her slacks and stretch. Encourage exercising the hands and arms by having the *person* brush his or her own hair or a caregiver's hair.

The 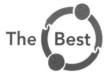 Best Friends Way

The Life Story: The more you know about a *person*, the easier it will be to incorporate moving and stretching into your daily routine. For instance, if the *person* has been a beautician, you can ask her to show you how to properly brush or comb her hair. If the *person* has been a baseball player, you can encourage him by talking about his good pitching arm as you prompt him to finish stretching into his sleeve.

Early Dementia: Encourage the *person* to be responsible for his or her personal care and help only when needed. Encourage the *person* to attend a physical fitness program or, if feasible, to have a personal trainer help him or her keep physically fit. Consider yoga for some *persons*.

Late Dementia: *Persons* who are chair or bed bound will benefit from basic range-of-motion exercises to prevent stiffness and improve comfort.

Music: Use music during personal care. Music encourages swaying and tapping of the feet.

Old Skills: Recall the school days when classes of calisthenics encouraged stretching and moving.

Conversation: Encourage, "Dollie, can you push your foot into the shoe? That's great, now go ahead and stretch your leg and move your ankle for some good morning exercise." Be positive during a bath, "Here is a nice soapy cloth to wash your feet." Share your feelings, "I like to try to touch the ceiling when I wake up in the morning. It feels so good." Reminisce, "Carter, did your cat, Pumpkin, always begin the day with a great stretch? Let's do the same thing."

An ounce of prevention...

Be sensitive to any medical limitations on moving and stretching.

The Basics

Dementia does affect sleep patterns, but here are some ideas that help.
- Maintain a routine; encourage going to bed at roughly the same time every night and make sure that the same steps are carried out leading up to bed.
- Allow for plenty of time to unwind and relax.
- Set the mood to be conducive for relaxing with low lighting, little noise, or a favorite song or video.

Planning Tip: Keeping a *person* physically active, stimulating him or her through rich activities, and encouraging time spent out of doors will help a *person* feel tired and sleep more soundly.

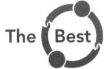

The (Best) Friends Way

Life Story: What has been the *person's* routine and life-long habit regarding going to bed? Is he or she a late-night *person* or an early-to-bed *person*? Did he or she have certain rituals they performed before going to bed (i.e., reading, bathing, sipping hot milk)? If so, make sure to incorporate those into the routine of going to bed.

Music: Use soft music or relaxation tapes to calm down and unwind from the day.

Old Sayings: "Early to bed, early to rise, makes a man (or woman) healthy, wealthy, and wise."

Sensory: Enjoy the softness of flannel or satin pajamas. Feel the coolness of the sheets as you crawl into bed on a hot summer night.

Spirituality: Many *persons* closed the day with a prayer, a reading, a favorite song, or a poem. Others may have shared the day's experiences with a special someone. Be attentive to a *person's* need to maintain as much of a normal life as possible.

Conversation: Use light conversation to cue the *person* of the hour, "I'm beginning to get quite sleepy, are you?" Reminisce, "Judy, remember in the old farmhouse, before we had heat, we would pile lots of blankets on the bed at night? Boy, were those heavy!" Share your past, "I recall my father always reading me a bedtime story. Would you like to read some poems together?"

Going to Bed

Do you have pleasant thoughts about going to bed: a comfortable mattress, soft sheets, or your favorite pillow? Bedtime is some individuals' favorite time of day! In the face of dementia, going to bed can often seem like a difficult and daunting task. With help, *persons* with dementia can re-experience these positive feelings.

Waking Up

Do you jump out of bed each morning or struggle to crawl out from under the covers? Everyone has a routine and preferences for waking up that help to set the tone for the day. *Persons* with dementia will benefit from a good start in the morning.

The Basics

It is best to let the *person* wake up without prompting. If you need to wake the *person* up, call his or her name, introduce yourself, and gently touch the *person* to wake him or her. Allow for plenty of time. If the *person* feels rushed, he or she will feel anxious—a feeling that may stay around for the rest of the day. Establish a routine for each morning.

The 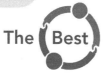 Best Friends Way

Life Story: Know the *person's* preferences regarding waking up. Did the *person* jump into the shower first thing in the morning or prefer to take some time waking up over a cup of coffee? Has the *person* always been a late sleeper or did he or she rise early? Does the *person* want to look at the paper right away before getting dressed? Know what the *person* prefers to drink in the morning: coffee, tea, something else. Also, know how they take their tea or coffee: black, with sugar, or with milk or cream.

Exercise: Encourage the *person* to stretch and take a deep breath to get ready for the day.

Humor: Beginning the day with light kidding and joking can set a pleasant tone and put everyone in a good mood.

Music: If the *person* responds well, sing a song such as "Wake with the Buttercups" or "Beautiful Morning."

Sensory: A gentle, reassuring touch may be a wonderful way to stir someone from sleep. Make certain someone's hearing aids, eyeglasses, and dentures are in place so that he or she can connect with the physical environment.

Spirituality: Some *persons* like to start the day with a prayer or meditation.

Conversation: Gently orient the *person*, "Good morning Margaret. It's going to be a wonderful Tuesday." or "It's Sunday. Let's get ready for church." Provide a choice, "Would you like your eggs fried or scrambled this morning?" Reminisce, "Remember when you had to go gather the eggs each morning?" Connect with the *person*, "Dr. Thomas, I'm glad you're wide awake, I need someone to talk to."

An ounce of prevention...

The way a person is greeted upon waking up can often determine how he or she greets the day.

CHAPTER SEVEN

Especially for Men

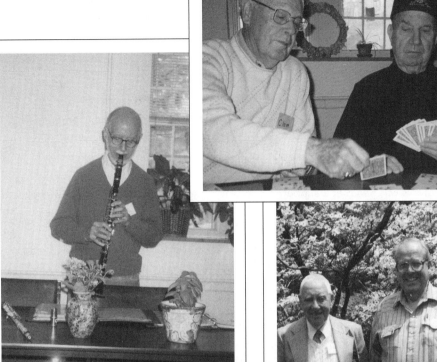

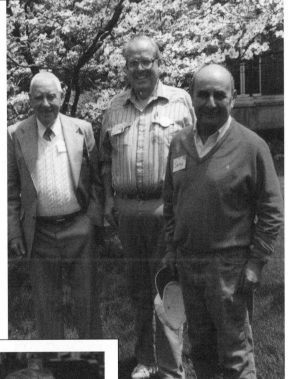

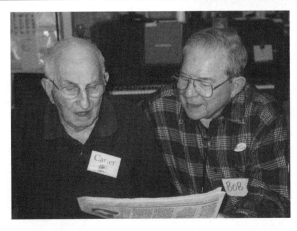

Especially for Men

Many older men devoted much of their early years to work and making money, engaging in few, if any, recreational activities. Staff members in long-term care programs often hear the following refrain when asking men to join activities, "I'm much too busy for that" or "I've got to work today." However we analyze it, men provide a greater challenge to activities professionals.

An example of this was heard at a support group when a son complained to us about the activities at his father's dementia unit, "My dad just isn't interested in the crafts or group programs. He needs to do more guy things!"

Although it seems politically incorrect to title a chapter this way, activities staff members sympathize with this son—they, too, are looking for more "guy things," activities especially for men.

The generation of men who have dementia today is made up of many individualists. Many took part in group activities through sports or service clubs, but others spent more time in solitary activities and hobbies. Many of us have heard the familiar refrain, "My dad was never a joiner!" Making matters worse, men often do not enjoy arts-and-crafts projects, which tend to dominate traditional activity programs.

With the caution that everyone is different (many women may enjoy the following activities and some men won't), this chapter presents activities that are designed especially for men. They include some obvious topics such as *Sports* (see page 137) and *Cars* (see page 138), but also some activities associated with military service (see page 142) and handling money (see page 148). Some of the activities in this chapter can be done in class or group settings. Others can be built around one-to-one times. *The Men's Club* involves creating a special space or time where men can come together and enjoy a morning coffee or a special program (see page 150). For this generation, many clubs were same sex (e.g., men's social clubs, men's military retiree groups). Having a special place or club might encourage a reluctant *person* to participate in group activities.

Throughout the chapter are ideas about how to talk to men about activities. Communicating with knack (for example, asking for help, encouraging, and tying activities to the *person's* work-related past) is important in order to get men to try new things.

With societal changes, we guess that future generations will see fewer differences in activity programming between men and women, but for now, "vive la difference!"

CHAPTER SEVEN ACTIVITIES

The Basics

- Sports magazines, uniforms, sports equipment, old trophies, and old photos
- The daily sports page

Watch a sporting event, whether you attend one or just view it on television. Play a guessing game of the names of sports teams.

Don't be afraid to engage in athletic activities, this can help keep the *person* active and provide an opportunity to exercise during the day. Examples include tossing a ball, kicking a ball, indoor putting with a golf club, and going to a golf driving range.

Variations: Create a sports bar or club atmosphere with a pool table and nonalcoholic beer. The Internet is a rich source of sports trivia and statistics.

Sports

Many men are avid sports fans. *Persons* with dementia often remain physically robust, and they may keep their long-held interest in sports. This activity celebrates sports, ranging from being an active participant to being an "armchair" athlete.

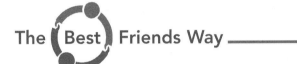

The (Best) Friends Way

Life Story: Focus on the *person's* sport of choice. Did he play a particular sport? Are there any sports he enjoys watching? Has he received any special awards or trophies from playing sports? Is he from a city or state known for a particular sport or sports team?

Humor: Sporting events can be a prime time for funny happenings (a terrible golf shot or missing an easy goal). Don't be afraid to make fun of yourself, if you don't know anything about the sport or if you're clumsy when you try to play!

Early Dementia: Men may enjoy continuing to participate in a biking or hiking group.

Music: Sing a college team's "fight song" or "Take Me Out to the Ballgame."

Old Sayings: "Catch it on the fly." "Hitting a home run."

Old Skills: *Persons* often retain good hand–eye coordination that helps them continue some sporting activities.

Sensory: Examine a collection of balls used for various sports, see them, touch them, and identify them (e.g., pigskin football, polo ball, softball, Ping-Pong ball).

Conversation: Ask an easy question, "Do you like baseball or football the most?" Ask an opinion, "I like the Detroit Pistons. Do you?" Reminisce, "Did you ever coach a team? What do you think makes a good coach?" Honor the life story, "What kind of uniform did you wear for that sport? What type of equipment did you use?" While watching a football game, "John, what did you think of that play?"

An ounce of prevention...

Be careful that sports equipment is not thrown or hit in a way that might be harmful to others in the room.

Cars

Do you remember your first automobile—whether you saved and bought it new or got an old family hand-me-down? Men especially seem to have a fascination with cars. Men with dementia may retain this interest and enjoy talking about and looking at cars.

The Basics

- Automobile magazines, new car brochures, and books on cars
- Car parts and tools

Internet keywords include: vintage cars, manufacturer web sites, and car clubs. Look through automotive magazines for pictures of cars, especially those that focus on vintage cars. Talk about the change in the price of cars since he bought his first car. You can also encourage the *person* to handle car parts and tools for fixing cars, visit a new car lot, or collect glossy new car brochures.

Variations: If available, have an old car to tinker with! Many men enjoy sitting in a car.

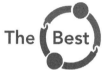

The (Best) Friends Way

Life Story: How did the *person* learn to drive? Did he work as a mechanic or fix his own cars? Did he sell cars or work in an auto-related industry? Reminisce about his first car. Did he learn to drive at age 13 on a farm or later in life at age 30 because he lived in a city with subways and buses? Did he ever travel by car cross-country?

Exercise: Washing a car together expends lots of energy!

Humor: Joke about students who try to get 19 people inside a small Volkswagen "Bug."

Early Dementia: Attend a meeting of a vintage car club or go to a special automobile event.

Late Dementia: Going for a ride, parking, and simply sitting in the car and looking out over a beach or activities in a park can provide a pleasurable activity.

Music: There are many songs themed around cars including commercial jingles such as, "In my Merry Oldsmobile" or "See the USA in Your Chevrolet."

Sensory: Riding in a car with the windows down and smelling the fresh air can bring back great memories.

Conversation: Together, see how many cars you can name from the 1930s, 1940s, 1950s, or even more recent cars. Reminisce, "Do you remember when cars had rumble seats?" or "Did cars always have air conditioning and seat belts?" Ask for advice, "How do you change the oil in a car?" Share a mutual interest, "Did you ever have a 'dream' car—one that you always wanted but never could get? Was it a Corvette? A convertible?"

An ounce of prevention...

Be aware of the possibility that the person may be sad or angry about having to give up driving. Focus on the cars, not driving.

138

The Basics

Create a space where a staff member can pull out tools and work with *persons* on common activities. Organize an old toolbox while examining the tools (e.g., hammer, screwdriver, pliers, lathe) and discussing each one.

Look at antique tools and guess what they are used for (e.g., a froe—a cleaving tool for splitting shingles). Use some of the tools you've discussed to make something or do a simple repair. Ask him to help you tighten a screw, clamp something tight, or hammer a nail.

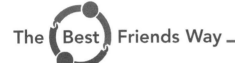

The Best Friends Way

Life Story: Many men have collected tools and may enjoy showing them to you. Was he a "Mr. Fix-It" around the home? Did he work in an occupation using tools? How was his toolbox organized—was everything thrown together or did everything have its proper place?

Humor: Joke about the funny names for some tools such as "monkey wrench" and "needle-nose pliers." Share humorously, "I can't tell you what I said when I accidentally hit my thumb with the hammer!"

Early Dementia: Making a simple repair, hanging up a picture, or helping with a project can build self-esteem. Visit a local hardware store and browse.

Old Sayings: "He hit the nail on the head." "Tools of the trade."

Sensory: The smell of sawdust, the cool feel of iron, the sound of sandpaper against the wood, or the brightly colored handles of tools are all sensory rich.

Conversation: Ask for information, "What do you use this tool for?" Reminisce with some humor, "Do you remember the tools we used before power tools? How did you drill without a power drill?" Ask an easy question, "Mark, can you ever have enough tools?" Share some of your own successes and failures building or fixing things.

Tools of the Trade

A workshop can be a wonderful place for building and fixing things, or simply to escape from the demands of the day. Men with dementia may enjoy handling tools and using them to fix and build things or to just "fool around" in the workshop.

An ounce of prevention...

Make a careful assessment of the person's cognitive and physical skills and match these to an appropriate level of involvement with this activity.... Take particular care with power tools; at some point a man with dementia will no longer be able to manage once-familiar tools.

Scrap Wood Sculpture

Some of the most famous sculptors have been men. This is a good art project for men with dementia who like to do things with their hands because it provides an opportunity to combine old skills with familiar materials and an opportunity for creative expression.

The Basics

- Scrap wood pieces small enough to hold in your hand
- Sandpaper
- Nails (appropriately sized to nail together pieces of the scrap wood)
- Wood glue
- Hammers
- Spray paint
- Newspapers to cover work area

Sand the pieces of wood to smooth the rough edges. Sanding becomes a preliminary part of the work and can be done as an activity in itself. Select a piece of scrap wood to become the foundation of the sculpture, perhaps the largest piece. Arrange the wood pieces in interesting ways on the base. Nail in place (or glue if the pieces are small enough) one by one until you have completed a unique sculpture. Let the glue dry. Spray paint all one color to add elegance and interest.

Variations: Glue on three-dimensional collage items before sculpture is spray-painted. Add hand-painted detail after the spray paint is dry.

The 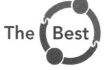 Best Friends Way

Life Story: Has the *person* ever worked with wood? He might know the right size nails to use or how to glue the pieces together. He may tell you about the experiences he has had with wood in the past.

Early dementia: Accompany these men to an adult education class on sculpting. Many men with dementia rediscover their creativity.

Late Dementia: A *person* may enjoy just holding a piece of wood.

Old Skills: Hammering, driving nails, sanding, and painting are all old skills.

Sensory: Look at and feel the textures of the wood, smell it. Enjoy the sounds of hammering.

Conversation: Discuss the type of wood you think it might be. Reminisce, "The grain of the wood on this piece reminds me of my mother's dining room table." Ask an opinion, "Is oak or pine better for building furniture?" Ask for information, "Jack, what is the hardest kind of wood?" Plan together, "Shall we build it to stand tall or to lay flat?" Be ambitious, "Let's build something we can display at an art gallery or in the courtyard of the day center!"

An ounce of prevention...

Use only one hammer for the activity. It will be easier to monitor for safety. Keep your eyes on the nails.

The Basics

Caregivers with knack understand the importance of work to most men. Celebrate his occupation or work life by gathering items he might have used in his work, such as a stethoscope, tape measure, or hard hat to spark memories. Talk and reminisce with him about his occupation or the various jobs he has held. Consider setting up an "office" or desk with familiar items and papers.

Occupations

Work occupies much of our lives and is tied to long-held values of being productive. For a man with dementia, creative activities related to work can help diminish feelings that he's "not worth anything" and help him feel pride and a sense of accomplishment.

The 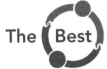 Best Friends Way

Life Story: Learn what you can about his occupation—equipment used, special training needed, exactly what he did. Does he have any particular achievements or aspects of his occupation that he is proud of? Note any titles associated with his work (e.g., Foreman, Labor Secretary, Doctor, Colonel). Ask questions specifically related to his field: "Would you have given me a loan?" to a bank officer. Did he belong to a labor union?

Music: Sing in a light-hearted fashion, "I've Been Working on the Railroad" while working together.

Old Sayings: "Don't put off until tomorrow what you can do today." "Breadwinner." "Daily grind." "Business before pleasure."

Spirituality: Some individuals view their chosen line of work as more than a job—it is a "calling." Discuss this concept and how a calling is different from a job.

Conversation: Ask an easy question, "Were you all work and no play? What does that old saying mean?" Seek more information, "Tell me about your work. How did you choose it as your job?" Provide a cue to start a discussion, "Blaine, was it hard to sleep during the day when you worked at night?" Ask about an early memory, "I hear you are a journalist. Is it true that they used to pay you per word for your stories?" Honor the life story, "Did you follow in your father's footsteps?"

An ounce of prevention...

Be aware that a person may be offended if you talk about his work in the past tense; he may still consider himself a banker, rancher, teacher, cook, or salesman even if not currently active.... Some men become anxious if you talk to them about work; they get confused about past and present and may worry that they are late for work!

Military

Many men have been in military service of their country, whether it was for a short period of time or as a career choice. *Persons* with dementia may enjoy talking about their military experience, which for many is the defining experience of their lives.

The Basics

Gather information and trivia about military life. (Internet keywords: World War II, Liberty Bonds, Meatless Monday, Daylight Savings Time, Army, Navy, Marines, Air Force, Coast Guard.) Find pictures of military life, including uniforms and insignias.

Look for items that might spark memories of enlisted days such as Air Force wings or an Army handbook. Discuss the information with a group of men or one-to-one. Include trivia questions you've gathered from your research.

The (Best) Friends Way

Life Story: Learn about his service in the military. Find out what branch he served in, his rank, if he traveled, and what his job was. Did he receive any special awards of merit or medals? Was the military his career? Was he in the National Guard? Does he recall his early days as a draftee? Was his military experience positive or traumatic? What kind of plane did he fly in World War II, Korea, or Vietnam?

The Arts: Make a scrapbook of the *person's* life in the military or enjoy looking at one already created.

Humor: Laugh together, "I had two left feet when I was trying to march." Read old or current Beetle Bailey comic strips.

Early Dementia: Encourage the *person* to attend military reunions or social clubs related to his military service.

Music: Sing patriotic songs and songs for each branch of service (Air Force, Army, Navy, Marines).

Old Sayings: "Hurry Up and Wait." "Uncle Sam Wants You."

Sensory: Looking at pictures about the military, handling shiny belt buckles or dog tags, or even shining shoes can evoke memories of military life.

Conversation: Ask for information, "What is a tour of duty? Did anyone ever go on one?" Introduce some humor, "Tell me about your training at boot camp. Do you think I'd make it in a boot camp?" or "Did you ever have KP duty?" Reminisce, "What type of uniform did you wear? When did you wear your 'dress blues'?" Tease, "Mark, let me see your crisp salute."

An ounce of prevention...

Keep the emphasis on aspects of military life such as uniforms, training, and travel. Avoid discussions of combat, which could be upsetting to the person or to others listening in.

The Basics

Make a careful assessment of the *person's* cognitive and physical skills and match these with an appropriate activity ranging from working in a shop with supervision, to whittling, to just handling sandpaper and wood as part of a finishing process.

Discuss and look at tools related to woodworking such as a lathe or auger. Look at different types of wood. Work on a simple woodworking project such as building a sandbox for children or a bird feeder (see page 79) or help assemble a precut bookcase. Men may enjoy looking at one of the many magazines devoted to this hobby.

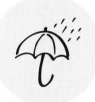

Woodworking

Many men study, practice, enjoy, and become quite accomplished at woodworking. Men with dementia enjoy practicing long-held skills like woodworking and may be able to continue the hobby with assistance.

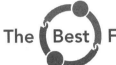

The (Best) Friends Way

Life Story: If his hobby is woodworking, enjoy his past creations! Look at them together and let him tell you how he made each one. Does he have special woodworking tools that are heirlooms? Ask him to tell you about them. Find out if he was "handy" in general with tools or carpentry; discuss this even if he was not specifically a woodworker himself.

The Arts: Create a carved or whittled object for all to enjoy.

Humor: Try to say, "How much wood could a woodchuck chuck if a woodchuck could chuck wood."

Early Dementia: Plan and design a project together, or encourage him to enroll in a class or workshop. Buddy up with a staff member or other family member who woodworks to keep the hobby going and provide some supervision.

Late Dementia: Hold and admire a finished piece.

Sensory: Sand the wood and feel the surface to see if it is smooth. Smell the different types of wood. Notice the changes of color throughout a piece of wood.

Conversation: Ask an easy question, "What is whittling? Have you ever whittled?" Start a discussion, "Mike, how did you learn woodworking? Did someone teach you or did you teach yourself?" Honor the life story, "Have you ever made a piece of furniture?" or "Is it true that you carved duck decoys?" Ask an opinion, "What is the best type of wood to work with?"

An ounce of prevention...

This is a good one-to-one activity that can use up a lot of pent-up energy, but pay attention to safety concerns around sharp objects.

Trains

Trains are a common form of transportation in many parts of the country, and many men may have traveled for business or taken their families on vacation via train. Men with dementia may retain a fascination for trains, and this activity can spark a good one-to-one discussion or a larger, classroom discussion with great success.

The Basics

Look for information and trivia on trains in books or on the Internet. (Internet keywords: trains, train schedules, steam locomotion, model trains, Trans-Siberian Railroad, or Orient Express.) Collect items that relate to trains such as a conductor's hat, train schedules, a train whistle, or a signal lantern. Use this information and props to spark discussion and to create a list of trivia questions.

Create a train room with a donated or borrowed train set. Visit a nearby train museum or train station. Review old train schedules or look at maps indicating train routes.

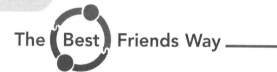

The (Best) Friends Way

Life Story: Has he worked on a train? Has he traveled by train for business or pleasure? Did he live near railroad tracks? Was he an engineer who might understand and know about building a railroad bridge across a chasm? Was he a free spirit, hitching a ride or "jumping" on a train car? Was there a train station in his hometown? Is he a model train buff?

The Arts: Find and read poems or short stories about trains (e.g., Emily Dickinson's *I Like to See it Lap the Miles*).

Humor: Joke about running to catch a train.

Early Dementia: Take a train ride and enjoy the sights and sounds of the day. In some cities, a ride on a "light rail" or "commuter" train may make for a pleasant outing. In some places, a train trip with a dinner car can be a fun short trip.

Music: Sing the song, "Chattanooga Choo-Choo."

Sensory: The sound of a train whistle can bring back fond memories. Holding a miniature train and feeling the metal can be pleasurable.

Conversation: Reminisce, "Tell me about your first train ride. Where did you go?" Try to recall the professions that work on a train (porter, conductor, or engineer). Ask for information, "Lewis, where is Grand Central Station? Have you ever been there?" Share your story, "I don't think I could sleep on a train, could you? Did you ever sleep in a Pullman car?" Dream together, "Wouldn't it be fun to ride on the Orient Express?"

The Basics

Collect information and trivia about old radio shows, stars, and characters. (Internet keywords: old-time radio, *Fibber McGee & Molly*, *Amos & Andy*, *Bob Hope & Jack Benny*.) Listen to and discuss recordings of old radio shows or to "oldie" shows on the radio today. Find an old-fashioned radio that still works and enjoy tuning it together. Read aloud an old radio script. Try to mimic or figure out how early radio programmers created sound effects!

Subscribe to satellite or cable digital radio stations if your budget allows. The selection of programs is enormous.

Variation: Study and look at all of the various types of modern radios including novelty ones (for example, radios in a ceramic bear or inside a pen).

Radio

Radio was the major source of news and entertainment in the days before television. Many men remember their favorite programs on the radio. Recordings of radio programs may spark memories and continue to provide entertainment for men with dementia.

The 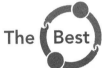 Best Friends Way

Life Story: Learn about his favorite radio shows. Was he a radio operator, or did he ever build a radio set? Did he depend on the radio for a weather report? Did he ever operate a CB radio or enjoy ham radio? Did he listen to radio in the car during a long commute to work? Would he enjoy programming in Spanish? Did he ever listen to the BBC on short-wave radio?

Humor: Listen to recordings of old radio comedies.

Music: Find a good oldies or jazz station, and turn it up.

Sensory: Feel the vibration of the bass sounds on a radio's speakers.

Spirituality: Talk about how religious programs have been and are still popular on the radio.

Conversation: Discuss the famous *War of the Worlds* show by Orson Welles, (a live radio broadcast in 1938 of a fictional tale about an invasion from Mars that many thought was real, causing a panic). Did anyone hear it? Reminisce, "Did you have a radio at home? When did you listen to it?" Recall historic events, "What president started the first fireside chats?" (FDR). Confer, "Did you use the radio for news?" Share stories about historical events they may have heard for the first time on the radio.

Flags

The flag is a national symbol that we have been taught to respect and honor. Flags also have symbolic meaning from countries to states to regiments or even organizations and clubs. Men with dementia may have a deep respect for the flag and enjoy handling, discussing, or "raising" the flag each day.

The Basics

Go to books or the Internet for information, images, and trivia about flags. (Internet keywords: flags, Betsy Ross, flag etiquette, nautical flags.) Collect flags from various locales. Print photographs from the web of flags of the states, of countries, and of nautical flags and discuss their histories. Use this information for a class discussion or for a one-to-one conversation. Flag etiquette (e.g., not touching the ground, when to raise and take it down, folding flags) remains fascinating for many men.

The 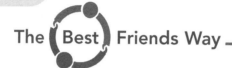 Friends Way

Life Story: Research the flag of his home state or country. Would he consider himself particularly patriotic? Identify flags that relate to the *person's* life. Did he enjoy watching the Olympics? Talk about the "Parade of Flags" or opening ceremony. Was anyone a sailor who learned the meaning of various nautical flags?

The Arts: Make a flag using torn paper art (see page 58). Create flags from the birth countries of men in the group.

Music: Proudly sing, "You're a Grand Old Flag," "The Star Spangled Banner," or a home state song.

Old Sayings: "Flag me down." "Raising a red flag." "Flag man."

Sensory: Admire colors of the flags. If you have flags to show, feel the fabric. Hear the sound of a flag flapping in the breeze.

Conversation: Play a trivia game, "How many red stripes and white stripes are on the United States flag?" or "How are the stars lined up?" Tap an old memory, "Who designed or sewed the first United States flag?" Ask for advice, "How should the flag be displayed?" Recall an early memory, "Did you say the Pledge of Allegiance before school classes?" Share information, "In 1958, the United States flag only had 48 stars. What 2 states were added to make up the 50 stars we have today?" (Alaska & Hawaii—1959) Inquire, "Alex, you are from Calgary. Why is there a maple leaf on Canada's flag?"

An ounce of prevention...

Be certain that all staff understand that flags have highly symbolic value and need to be treated with respect. Also note that not everyone present may be a United States citizen, so be respectful of differences.

The Basics

Gather information and trivia about the weather from books or the Internet to use in discussions. (Internet keywords: weather, meteorology, weather records, Groundhog Day.)

Read the daily forecast and study a weather map in the newspaper (look at local weather as well as the weather around the world). Men enjoy gadgets, so look into getting an indoor/outdoor thermometer, a barometer, a weather vane, a windsock, or a rain gauge. Enjoy looking at and discussing the weather forecasts in *Farmer's Almanac*.

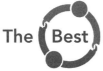

The Best Friends Way

Life Story: Did his job depend on the weather, such as construction work? Are his hobbies outdoors, and do they involve watching the weather? Did he farm or garden outdoors? Were there any traumatic experiences associated with weather such as a major storm, or a hurricane, or a tornado? What kind of climate did he grow up in? Did someone have a talent for predicting the weather?

Humor: Chuckle about the time you and your family got drenched during a picnic.

Early Dementia: A man may find meaning in being in charge of clipping weather reports from the paper daily or checking the outside rain gauge or indoor barometer and posting the information daily on the bulletin board. He can read the weather report aloud each day over breakfast.

Music: Play recordings of "April Showers," "Raindrops Keep Falling on My Head," and "In the Good Old Summertime."

Old Sayings: "Raining cats and dogs." "Weather will be weather, whether or not." "It's raining, it's pouring, the old man is snoring."

Sensory: Go outside more often, even if the weather isn't perfect. Seeing nature at work is the ultimate sensory experience.

Conversation: Celebrate, "Doesn't the sun feel good and warm on our shoulders? What a beautiful day!" Speculate with a person living in Arizona, "Do you miss the four seasons?" Use the life story, "Jim, didn't you travel to Florida every winter to escape the cold?" Have a laugh, "I think we can predict the weather better than that television forecaster!" Ponder, "Does the groundhog really foretell the weather?"

Weather

Weather influences the daily lives of all of us. Many men with dementia enjoy predicting the weather and talking about its impact on daily life.

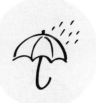

An ounce of prevention...

Be cautious that bad weather doesn't evoke anxiety or fear. For example, if a storm is coming, a staff member can smile to calm fears and note that rain is good for the crops, flowers, and lawn!

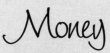
Money

Everyone has used money throughout their lives. Because money is something almost all men have thought a lot about, worried about, and worked for, money remains of interest for a man with dementia.

The Basics

Discuss values around money (e.g., saving versus spending). Talk about their first jobs and salaries. Collect foreign and historic money (coins and bills) to show to the group. Talk about current money. See if they can remember the artwork on each bill. Look at old catalogs and talk about prices then and now. Share superstitions about money, such as a lucky penny, throwing coins in a fountain, or keeping the first dollar bill that comes in from a business.

Variation: Discuss items used throughout history as currency such as tobacco, corn, wheat, salt, nails, silver, gold, beads, and shells.

The 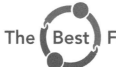 Best Friends Way

Life Story: How did he earn his first dollar? You can use foreign money to discuss an individual's heritage or favorite trips. What was his family's value concerning money? Does he always carry a wallet or billfold with money, or did he carry a money clip?

The Arts: Make rubbings of coins (see Lace Rubbings, page 183).

Humor: Joke (or humorously cry) over income taxes.

Early Dementia: Caregivers with knack help a *person* maintain his independence as long as possible. Give some assistance, when needed, in helping the person continue to have some involvement with his finances—record keeping, filing, keeping the check register, or reviewing statements are all options. A man may also enjoy "giving advice" to others about money management, investments, or major purchases.

Late Dementia: A man may enjoy counting money or carrying his wallet with a few dollar bills inside.

Old Sayings: "A penny saved is a penny earned." "Penny pincher." "Penny wise and pound foolish." "Money to burn." "Flip a coin." "Easy come, easy go."

Sensory: Enjoy the feeling of coins in the hand, hearing the sounds of change jingling, and seeing colorful foreign currency.

Conversation: Ask for advice, "Do you think it's better to buy a new car or used car?" Ask an opinion, "I paid 3 dollars for this loaf of bread. Don't you think that's expensive?" Discuss a past trip, "Have you ever traveled to a U.S. Mint?" Be philosophical, "Does money make a man happy?" Discuss today's prices of cars, houses, and groceries—are they outrageously high or just right?

An ounce of prevention...

Exercise caution because some persons may worry about where their own money is, or if they have enough cash on hand to "pay" for their lunch.

The Basics

Make a daily newspaper available for a man to read by himself or with assistance. If you read the paper together, talk about the headlines. Discuss how a paper is produced or printed. Look through the advertisements to discuss how things have changed, all the new inventions and the increased prices. Read the sports pages together. If someone is interested, track his daily horoscope.

Training Tip: The national newspaper *USA Today* is a particularly good source of colorful news bites and trivia, outstanding sports coverage, state-by-state news, and weather.

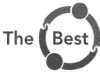 The **Best** Friends Way

Life Story: Tie articles in the newspaper to his life story. Look for particular events he remembers or gather newspapers from his hometown. Has he ever been featured in a newspaper story? Get a copy of the article and reminisce. Did he have a newspaper delivery route? Is his morning ritual a cup of coffee and a newspaper?

Humor: There may be a funny story or photograph that will spur your laughter. Read the comics together; reminisce about characters in some of the classic comic strips such as "Peanuts" and "Blondie."

Late Dementia: The person may enjoy being with you while you read and comment on the paper.

Sensory: The feel and smell of newsprint may bring back lots of memories. Reading the newspaper and enjoying the first cup of coffee of the day often go together.

Spirituality: Read the religious section from a newspaper. Look at lists of churches or services and discuss.

Conversation: Reminisce, "Roy, what did houses sell for in the 1960s?" Ask an easy question, "What section do you always read first?" Look at the different prices of things in the ads and talk about whether that is a fair price to pay. Share sports trivia and ask about favorite teams. Comment, "I always read the funnies first. Do you?"

Newspapers

Reading the newspaper is a favorite pastime for many men. Men with dementia may no longer be able to fully read, comprehend, and retain a newspaper story, but they may relate to the symbolic value of handling a paper and staying "current."

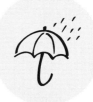

An ounce of prevention...

For a person with dementia, a little worry may grow into a big one. Screen out troubling news when possible.

The Men's Club

Some men enjoy going to regular meetings of veteran's groups, service clubs, or coffee at McDonald's or a neighborhood restaurant each morning. This activity involves creating a special space or time of day for a "men's gathering" or "club" that men with dementia can call their own.

The Basics

Come up with a creative name for a daily meeting for men (e.g., Eagle's Club, Quarterback's Club). Schedule a regular meeting time and place. Create a pleasurable atmosphere with refreshments, comfortable seating, good lighting, a pool table, a putting green, and newspapers.

Encourage a male staff member to participate and lead a discussion, or at least facilitate. Consider electing "officers" of the daily group and creating membership cards. Build in a daily ritual, pouring coffee in the morning or having a nonalcoholic cocktail hour each afternoon.

Variation: A similar society can be created for women! The club could also go on outings as a group or take on a community charitable project.

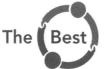

The Best Friends Way

Life Story: Consider if any of the men have been in clubs before. Decorate the room with themes from the men's lives (e.g., the stock market, hobbies, college football). Consider putting up pictures of the members on the wall with a brief note about each *person.*

Humor: Have posted a joke-of-the-day or present to members a humorous take on the day's news.

Early Dementia: Encourage a man to continue attending his service club meeting or other club social with a buddy or friend to help out.

Music: Have a good music system in the room and play music as an activity or in the background.

Spirituality: Discuss the bonds of friendship and how good it is to be together as a group of men supporting one another.

Conversation: Take pride in an achievement, "Good morning Mike, it's great to have you as a charter member of the club." Invite men whom you feel would benefit from the group, "Good morning Henry. I'm inviting you to go with me to the clubhouse." Tease, "I knew the smell of fresh coffee would get you in here!"

The Basics

Review past projects or hobbies of the *person*. Talk with him about the project or hobby and initiate some activity around it and see if the *person* responds. (For example, pull out the stamp collection and look at it together. See if the person shows interest and curiosity.) Help him complete just one step of the hobby. Sometimes just sorting through the supplies used for the hobbies is enjoyable.

Variation: Some men may have always had an interest in developing a new hobby but not an opportunity to move forward. It's good to try new things even after a *person* has been diagnosed with Alzheimer's disease.

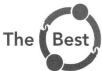

The (Best) Friends Way

Life Story: Make a detailed list of his hobbies and interests, including childhood activities. Talk to him about how he got started doing his hobby. Was he a collector of things such as antiques, political memorabilia, stamps, old tools, coins, or rocks? In a residential setting, you may find a number of men with common interests; match them up to enjoy their hobbies together.

The Arts: Create a display case to showcase a different *person's* hobby or collection each month.

Humor: Joke about unusual collections, such as a man with 10,000 books of matches.

Early Dementia: The *person* can continue most hobbies as usual with some specific cues to help when needed and some considerations taken for safety.

Late Dementia: If possible, have examples of the man's hobby displayed. If the *person* restored old cars, have a model car around or framed pictures of the cars.

Conversation: Let the *person* teach you, "I don't know much about bird watching. Where should we start?" Offer praise, "Uriel, I can't believe you created this beautiful wooden bowl. You are so talented!" Be surprised, "You collected all of these arrowheads?" Acknowledge the *person*, "You enjoy working with your hands, don't you? Your wood cabinets are beautiful."

Hobbies

Many of us have hobbies that provide hours of activity and purpose. With encouragement, adaptations, and adequate supervision, you can encourage men with dementia to continue finding satisfaction in stamp collecting, painting, woodworking, or any hobby the *person* practiced.

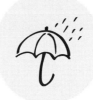

An ounce of prevention…

Sometimes reminders of a past hobby produce feelings of loss. Be accepting if the person *seems to have lost all interest in the hobby or doesn't remember it.*

CHAPTER EIGHT

In the Home

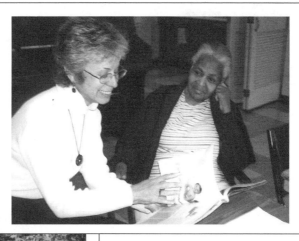

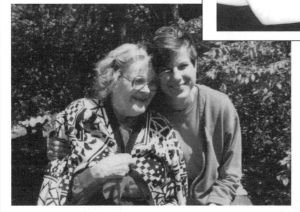

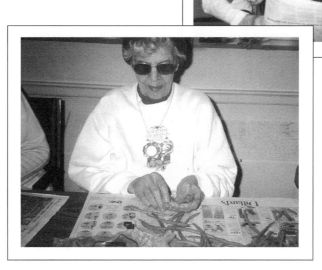

In the Home

Time spent in the home is usually treasured. For most of us, home is the favored place to be. It is where we start off and where we return. Most of us like to go other places, but there is nothing like getting back home. Home is the place where we rejuvenate and refresh ourselves, we eat and sleep, we replenish our spirit, and we rest. Home is a comfortable place to experience our feelings; we laugh, cry, pray, and act silly. If we are sick or tired, we want to be home. We celebrate our holidays and special times at home. We keep all of our possessions at home.

Home is the place where we do the things we enjoy the most. One of the most comfortable aspects of being at home is that we are generally free to choose our activities. Often, time at home is considered to be "free" time. Whether we rest, read, exercise, watch television, clean up, take a nap, cook, or work on our hobbies, it is our own time spent doing what we like. When we leave the house, we have specific places to go, errands to run, a job to do. At home there is the possibility for leisure.

It is common for persons with Alzheimer's disease to look for home, even when they are "home" and have lived in the same home all of their lives. When dementia progresses and this "home" cannot be found, the *person* needs reassurance and appropriate, meaningful things to do. *Persons* who have difficulty reasoning and remembering cannot always get the particular details correct about where they are, but they do long for the safe, comfortable feelings and activities of "home." A caregiver with knack designs activities in a home setting to evoke these happy moments.

The Best Friends approach to activities in the home is to take advantage of the positives, to turn everyday chores such as *Working Outside* (page 162) and *Laundry* (page 173) into meaningful activities. We also encourage participating in the community, being outdoors ,and taking short trips around the neighborhood (see *Taking a Drive*, page 163).

This chapter is especially helpful for home care providers and family caregivers. If you work in a residential or day center setting, peruse this chapter anyway. Our greatest goal is to make day and residential programs like home for *persons*. You may find inspiration in these activities, many of which can easily be adapted for other settings.

CHAPTER EIGHT ACTIVITIES

The Basics

Make sure the environment is conducive to reading (minimal distractions, good lighting), and be sensitive to vision disabilities/impairments or visual/spatial problems caused by dementia. Choose an upbeat reading from a book, a short story, a magazine, or a newspaper article. Adapt the activity to the person's remaining skills and interests. Keep the reading selections adult in nature, unless the *person* likes to reminisce and read or recite nursery rhymes with you. Take turns reading to each other if the *person* can read aloud.

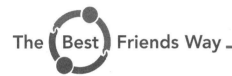

The (Best) Friends Way

Life Story: Tie a reading activity into the *person's* life story. Perhaps read from a family Bible, captions from photo albums, text of old postcards and greeting cards, or a treasured letter. Look through the business or sports section of a newspaper if those subjects are of interest to the *person*. Has the *person* enjoyed reading aloud to others, maybe children?

Early Dementia: Form your own book club! The caregiver and *person* can each read the same book or passage and then discuss it.

Late Dementia: Read to the *person* or enjoy quiet moments sitting together looking at picture books, photographs, or family albums.

Old Skills: Make this an intergenerational activity. Reading aloud to children is an old skill that can bring pleasure to all involved.

Sensory: The rhythmic sound of reading aloud or being read to can be soothing.

Spirituality: The *person* may find meaning through reading, or being read to, about nature, friendship, or selected religious texts.

Conversation: Reminisce, "You always read to your children when they were small, didn't you?" Ask an easy question, "Do you enjoy reading?" Use knack to encourage the activity, "I can't find my reading glasses. Would you read this newspaper story to me? I'm very interested in the topic." Admire a collection, "Silas, I'm so enjoying your collection of books. What are your favorites?"

Reading Together

Reading the morning newspaper, a good mystery novel, or an important new biography opens up a world of experiences and learning. The adaptations suggested in this activity may help a *person* with dementia continue to experience the joys of reading.

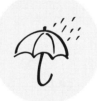

An ounce of prevention...

Note that some persons quickly forget the material due to their short-term memory loss and may become stressed if quizzed about the material.

Gardening

Gardening is a hobby many enjoy. Whether it is a few small pots or a larger flower or vegetable garden, this activity helps *persons* with dementia feel productive and provides wonderful flowers or food as a product of their labor!

The Basics

Establish a routine for work in the garden whether it is for planting new flowers and vegetables or maintaining an established garden. Select the time of day and length of time that is good for both the *person* and the caregiver. Choose plants that are familiar and easy to care for. Plan for safe access to the garden. Provide gentle prompts, demonstrate what needs to be done, and offer much praise when the *person* succeeds. If the *person* pulls up a flower, put it in a vase and enjoy it.

Variations: Care for potted plants or flowers inside. Make a terrarium with dirt, collected rocks, and tiny plants in a large jar or fish bowl. Plant tiny flower seeds, such as alyssum, in broken eggshells or an old china teacup.

Start a sweet potato vine by placing a sweet potato in a glass of water. Hold the sweet potato in place with toothpicks so it barely touches the water. The vine will grow out of the eyes of the sweet potato.

The 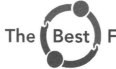 Best Friends Way

Life Story: Consider the *person's* background. Did he or she enjoy gardening around the home? Plant the *person's* favorite flower or vegetable. Does the *person* enjoy taking care of the garden tools, cleaning them up, and putting them in their proper place?

Late Dementia: Invite the *person* to sit outside and watch the gardening that is underway.

Old Skills: Weeding, watering, applying fertilizer, and picking vegetables are old skills that bring pleasure.

Sensory: Gardening is full of smells, sounds, touch, tastes, and visual feasts. Gardening involves putting hands into rich soil and even seeing an earthworm or two!

Conversation: Reminisce, "Dee, you had morning glories growing up your fence when you were a child, didn't you? What colors were they?" or "I remember that grandmother had tomatoes lined up on her window sill in the summer." Ask opinions, "Is this the right time of year to cut back the roses?" or "What color tulips should we plant this year?" Ask for advice, "Is this hole deep enough to plant this fruit tree?"

An ounce of prevention...

Be sure to use common-sense safety techniques around sharp tools. Keep your eye on the person to prevent wandering.

The Basics

Sweeping the floor is something almost everyone can do. To ensure success in this activity, give one direction at a time in a positive, simple manner while you show the *person* what you want. For example, hand the *person* a broom and say with a smile, "Would you mind sweeping up those crumbs on the floor for me, please?" Do not give the dust pan at the same time, it may confuse the *person*. Rather, hold the dust pan yourself and stay close by in case the *person* needs another prompt.

Variations: Be productive by mopping or vacuuming a floor.

A Clean Sweep

Some people take great pleasure in having squeaky-clean floors; others might have been more casual about housekeeping. Sweeping (indoors or outdoors) is an activity that almost everyone has done. It helps the *person* with dementia feel productive because it is a task that can be completed from beginning to end and one in which you see immediate results.

The 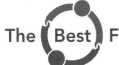 Best Friends Way

Life Story: Find out if the *person* did chores or housework, or if his or her partner did the job. Did the *person* grow up in a family that hired help? Did the *person* ever work as a housekeeper? Has the person been very meticulous about his or her surroundings? Does even a small scrap of paper on the floor bother the *person*?

Humor: "Too bad we can't ride this broom!"

Early Dementia: Maintain past routines and roles. It can be helpful to encourage someone to take on a particular household chore (such as keeping the patio swept). This helps the *person* feel that he or she is contributing to the household.

Late Dementia: Talk to the *person* while you do your work. Tell the *person* about what you know about how he or she used to clean. For example, "I know that you have always used a little bleach in your mop water."

Music: Sing "Whistle While You Work" from the movie *Snow White and the Seven Dwarves*.

Old Sayings: "This floor is so clean you could eat off it." "Many hands make light work." "A new broom sweeps clean." "Clean sweep."

Conversation: Talk about the way this work was done long ago. Discuss how brooms were once made by hand. Be humorous, "Did you ever know anyone who just swept the dirt out the front door?" Ponder, "How do they make brooms now?" Use humor, "Mr. Fong, I wish we had a dog that would eat the crumbs off of the floor. We could sit back and take it easy."

Washing Dishes

This activity can evoke old memories of doing the dishes with another family member. Some people dread the task and put it off; others won't go to bed without first washing every dish. Washing dishes builds bonds between the caregiver and *person* with dementia because it is an activity that two people can successfully do together—sharing the work as one washes and one dries.

The Basics

Invite the *person* to come to the kitchen sink, hand him or her one dirty dish, and ask, "Will you put this dirty dish in that water, please?" Wait for him or her to do so, and then hand over another dish with a similar verbal direction. Compliment and encourage the *person* along the way. Hand the *person* a wet dishcloth and say, "Will you swish this cloth around on that plate to get it clean, please?" Be ready to show what to do with the plate when it is clean (if the dishes are not clean, you can fix that later).

Variations: Ask the *person* to dry the dishes and stack them on the table so you can put them away. Have the *person* help you load the dishwasher.

The (Best) Friends Way

Life Story: Many people who have been parents will be able to talk about how they raised their children and whether they were strict with them about chores such as doing dishes. Did he or she have to take turns doing dishes when young? Did he or she ever bus tables or wash dishes in a restaurant?

Early Dementia: If the *person* enjoys washing dishes, he or she may want to be completely responsible for this task.

Music: This is a good time to listen to your favorite music in the background.

Old Sayings: "Cleanliness is next to godliness."

Sensory: Feel the warm water. Smell the clean soap. Admire how the dishes sparkle and shine when they are clean.

Conversation: Ask an easy question, "Don't you think there should be a better way to do dishes?" Reminisce, "Ruth, did your mother have pretty bone china plates. Were the dishes from England?" Discuss, "Do the dishes get cleaner when you put them in a dishwasher or when you wash them by hand?" Joke, "Did you ever leave a sink full of dishes? I have, and they were still there when I returned." Ask for information, "Why are some dishes called china?"

An ounce of prevention...

Switching to break-proof dishes can help the person participate in this activity longer, and relieve caregiver anxiety about breaking a good dish.

160

The Basics

Look for recipes of "one-dish" meals or dinners that can be prepared in 30 minutes or fewer. Purchase and set out ingredients ahead of time, then work together to start the meal. Focus on simple tasks. The *person* can break lettuce for a salad, stir spaghetti sauce, butter bread, and taste soup.

It is easier to keep the *person* engaged if meal preparation occupies only a short period of time.

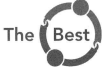

The (Best) Friends Way

Life Story: Did food play a role in the *person's* profession? What was his or her favorite food? Did he or she have a particular dish he or she was "famous" for (e.g., meatloaf, homemade fudge)? Learn if the *person* enjoyed cooking.

Humor: Joke about cooking disasters, like the time the poppy seed cake had no poppy seeds or the time you put too much cayenne pepper in a dish and everyone's taste buds were on fire!

Early Dementia: With some supervision, the *person* may still be able to prepare and organize meals.

Late Dementia: Gradually reduce the complexity of the task you offer as the disease progresses. Have the *person* taste the food, help you stir the batter, or hold the wooden spoon.

Old Skills: Cooking is an old skill for many. *Persons* may retain abilities to continue part of this activity with gentle help and encouragement.

Sensory: Aromas add to the anticipation of a cooked meal. Taste everything.

Conversation: Compliment, "I have always loved your meatloaf. You are such a good cook." Provide encouragement, "Continue the way you are stirring the soup. I can't wait to taste it!" Recognize the *person's* expertise, "Judy, you're a dietitian; do you think this big chocolate cake is good for us?" Use knack by showing you value the *person's* opinion, "Does this soup need a bit more salt?" Celebrate a person's heritage by preparing an ethnic dish (e.g., Matzo ball soup, chicken paprika, Korean barbecue).

Bon Appetit

Cooking is an art for many and a chore for others, but a necessary part of the day for most of us. The *person* with dementia can help with part of the meal or stay involved from beginning to end!

An ounce of prevention...

Employ common sense around sharp objects and hot surfaces.

Working Outside

It feels good to get outside and enjoy the fresh air and sunshine. Sunshine in moderate doses has health benefits for the body and can play a part in preventing depression. *Persons* with dementia can enjoy the outdoors and gain a feeling of accomplishment by doing simple yard tasks or tidying up a porch or patio.

The Basics

Choose a simple task to be done together. If raking leaves, get two rakes and demonstrate the raking of leaves into a pile.

Other outside chores include sweeping the porch or walk; picking up sticks; washing the car; picking fruit, berries, or vegetables; trimming shrubs; cleaning windows; or helping to build a trellis.

If the *person* has never been interested in working outside or is unable to, he or she may enjoy watching the work progress.

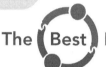

The Best Friends Way

Life Story: Know what outdoor tasks the *person* has previously done. He or she may be able to do these more easily than doing something new. Did the *person* spend a lot of time washing and waxing the car? Did he or she prefer working outside or inside?

Exercise: Being outdoors is a way to stay physically active.

Humor: Joke about the *person* being the director of activities if he or she is sitting on the side. Make a silly "snow person." Laugh about children jumping into a pile of leaves.

Old Skills: Hand–eye coordination often remains strong for such work as washing windows, raking, or filling the birdbath.

Sensory: The outdoors is incredibly sensory rich. Feel the cool breeze, see the beauty of nature, listen to the birds, touch the plants. Be sure to take plenty of breaks to soak it all in! Working outside can be a time to enjoy your own pets, to visit a friendly neighborhood cat or dog, or to have fun watching the acrobatics of squirrels.

Conversation: Enjoy the season, "Nan, look there are the daffodils peeking up from the ground. It must be spring!" Offer praise, "The house looks so pretty when the walk is swept clean! Thank you for doing that for me." Ask an opinion, "Mom, did I leave streaks on that window glass I cleaned?" Speculate, "I wonder where the term 'mother nature' came from?"

An ounce of prevention...

Always be there to provide support. Keep a watchful eye on the person *so that he or she does not get confused and walk away. If you have a gate, close it. Keep in mind that the* person *may have a short attention span and may only work for a few minutes.*

The Basics _____

Buckle up in the car and take a drive to a place where both of you can relax, away from heavy traffic areas. Stop at a coffee shop or ice cream parlor to share a treat. Park at a scenic place to enjoy the view from the car or take a nice stroll.

Often *persons* can run errands with their caregiver. This can be a win–win situation for both as caregivers have things to do and the *person* often wants to stay busy or be on the go.

The 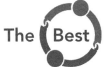 Best Friends Way _____

Life Story: Link *persons'* lifelong interests to your drive by taking them by places they might relate to, such as a golf course or a lake. Discuss past road trips. Use your time together in the car to reminisce about life and recall past cars that you have owned.

Humor: Chuckle while asking, "Should we go to Timbuktu?" Tease about having a poor sense of direction.

Late Dementia: Often a *person* will relax in the car during the late afternoon or early evening when restlessness or the desire to "go home" is strong.

Music: Listening to music in the car can add to the joy of the trip. Some *persons* love to sing in the car. Play a sing-along tape or CD or initiate the singing of a song.

Sensory: The quiet, enclosed space and the rhythm of the road seem to be soothing.

Spirituality: Being outdoors and seeing nature enriches the *person's* spiritual life.

Conversation: Observe, "Look at that new bridge going up. Have you ever seen such a big project?" Ask an opinion, "Do you think we should stay on the freeway or maybe explore a country lane?" Comment on the radio music, "Did your family argue about what station to listen to on long road trips?" Plant an idea, "I'm getting hungry. Would you like a hamburger for lunch?" Point out and read the traffic signs and billboards along the way.

Taking a Drive

Most of us are in our cars almost every day. Cars provide transportation, but they also represent freedom. *Persons* with dementia who are no longer driving often experience loss. A scenic drive can help address this loss.

An ounce of prevention...

Use the safety locks on the doors to ensure the person cannot open the door while riding. Avoid leaving the person in the car while you run an errand. Persons can get confused when they are left alone and often will get out of the car and become lost looking for you. (Enroll the person in the Alzheimer's Association's Safe Return program by visiting http://www.alz.org/SafeReturn or calling 1-800-272-3900.)

Shopping

Are you a shop-aholic, or do you know someone who is? *Persons* with dementia who have always been active and like to go places may continue to enjoy shopping trips if the atmosphere is light and easy. This activity has an added advantage of being one that care-givers often enjoy.

The Basics

Choose a time to shop when stores are not crowded. Think about the time of day when the *person* is at his or her best. Keep the shopping trip short to accommodate the *person's* attention span and stamina.

Become familar with the locations of unisex bathrooms. Assist the *person* as needed handling a wallet or purse.

Variations: Consider catalog shopping for *persons* who have trouble walking or who find going to a busy store overwhelming.

The 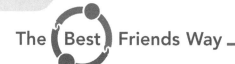 Best Friends Way

Life Story: Try different kinds of shopping, such as car dealerships, bookstores, and grocery stores. Link the type of shopping trips to a *person's* past interests. A woman who has enjoyed fashions may enjoy browsing at a dress shop. A man who enjoys fixing things may be happy in a hardware store.

Exercise: An indoor mall is a good way to get in a walk when the weather is bad.

Humor: Try on funny hats and sunglasses.

Early Dementia: The *person* may be able to do most activities associated with shopping if you provide some general support and supervision.

Music: Sing together "How Much Is that Doggy in the Window?"

Old Sayings: "Shop until you drop." "Window shopping."

Sensory: Go to a bookstore. Enjoy the comfortable, overstuffed chairs; a warm cup of coffee; or the soft background music while you people watch.

Conversation: Ask opinions, "Would this shirt look good on me?" Reminisce, "Addie, you used to shop for such a large family. That must have been a lot of work." Give a simple choice, "Do you like this dress in green or blue?" Ask advice, "What should I give May for her birthday?" Suggest, "Let's go to the sporting goods department and get some lures for our tackle box." Ask for an opinion, "What does it mean to go 'window shopping'?"

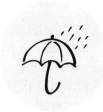

An ounce of prevention...

Be mindful of how the person is enjoying the trip, watching for increased confusion or other signs of stress. Carry a picture of him or her with you just in case he or she gets lost.

The Basics _____

If the person wants to make a call, have the name and number of the individual he or she is calling written down clearly or dial for him or her. If the call is for the *person*, announce the call to him or her, "Your sister, Susan, is on the phone and wants to talk with you!" Consider having friends and family members call on a schedule to build the connection into the *person's* weekly routine. Prompt callers as to the best topics for discussions and things to avoid.

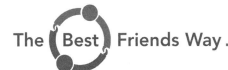

The (Best) Friends Way _____

Life Story: It is important to know the *person's* past attitudes about the telephone. Did he or she spend hours a day on the telephone chatting with friends, or keep every call short and sweet?

Humor: Joke about a *person* who used the telephone so much that "the receiver was attached to the ear."

Early Dementia: Look at new telephone products that have larger keypads, places for photographs that automatically dial a number, and enhanced volume control. These adaptations can help a *person* maintain his or her independence when using the telephone.

Late Dementia: Encourage family members to sing "Happy Birthday" to the *person* over the telephone.

Old Skills: Talking on the telephone with friends is an old skill not easily forgotten, but the *person* may get mixed up about the direction of the receiver and microphone or need assistance dialing.

Conversation: Just chit-chat, "How is the weather today?" Prompt the *person* to share the news about a new puppy the family has adopted. Honor the life story, "Mom, I'm baking a corn pudding using your special recipe." Reminisce about old-fashioned telephones, party lines, how telephones are different today than long ago. Ask opinions, "I am thinking about buying a new car, Dad, what do you think about a Buick?" or "I am having trouble with these kids. Didn't you have a good rule about raising children?"

Many people enjoy talking on the telephone. Families are often separated by distance, and the telephone is a wonderful way to keep in contact. Even though telephone use can become challenging for a *person* with dementia, many still want to stay in touch with friends and family.

An ounce of prevention...

Be careful to supervise telephone use for persons at home; unscrupulous telemarketers can prey on persons with dementia. Register the person on the national "Do Not Call" list.

165

Dining Out

Years ago most people cooked and ate the majority of their meals at home. Today, many people eat out frequently. Going out to eat can be a treat for the *person* with dementia and his or her caregiver.

The Basics

Consider the environment when choosing a restaurant. Choose a place that is not too noisy or crowded, has reasonably fast service, is accessible, and has a unisex bathroom. Going during off-peak hours is recommended; try a late breakfast or early dinner.

Many *persons* enjoy reviewing the menu but may need some prompting about their final order, "Mom, the salmon sounds good tonight. Would you like that?"

Become a "regular" at a specific restaurant or two. The restaurant staff will get to know you and may serve your needs better.

Planning Tip: Take something of interest for the person to enjoy while waiting for your meal or order a quick appetizer.

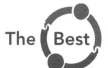

The (Best) Friends Way

Life Story: Know the *person's* likes and dislikes, favorite foods, and favorite restaurants. Plan ahead to talk about old stories or memorable meals in the past. Was the *person* a fast-food addict? Did he or she often eat in the car? Did he or she regularly have business lunches?

Early Dementia: *Persons* may enjoy maintaining their routine of going to a retired teachers lunch group.

Exercise: Take a walk before or after dinner.

Music: A restaurant with live music can be a treat for many *persons*.

Old Sayings: "My eyes were bigger than my stomach."

Sensory: Eating out makes way for aromas, tastes, textures, and music. Some places have extra visual appeal with fish tanks or fountains the *person* may enjoy.

Conversation: Ask opinions, "Did your mother make her flapjacks like this?" Give compliments, "You always make delicious pies. This is close but not as good as yours." Reminisce, "We used to go to the Sky View Diner to get the peach pie on Sunday evenings." Give a simple choice, "Would you like coffee or tea?"

An ounce of prevention...

Some caregivers like to have a written card to give the server, explaining that the person has Alzheimer's disease. It can explain any mistakes or inappropriate remarks that come.... Know when the time has come and the struggles of going out to eat outweigh the benefits.

The Basics _____

Research the kind of birds you want to attract to your backyard and the kind of seeds they eat. Survey the space around your home to find a good location that can be seen from your windows. Provide a bird feeder (see page 79), a birdbath, and a birdhouse. Plant bushes that grow berries to attract birds; incorporate the maintenance of the bird sanctuary into your everyday activities. Maintain a record of different birds sighted!

Variations: Plant a garden with plants that attract hummingbirds or butterflies (see Gardening, page 158).

(see page 79)

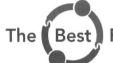

Creating a Bird Sanctuary

Creating a bird sanctuary is an ongoing activity that can be done with a friend. A bird sanctuary can be anything from one simple feeder to a corner of trees with many feeders, houses, and a birdbath. It can be effective for *persons* with dementia because it is meaningful, offers simple chores to do, and provides hours of entertainment.

The (Best) Friends Way _____

Life Story: Does the *person* enjoy nature? What does the *person* know about birds? Talk to the *person* about past homes he or she has lived in. Did he or she have birdhouses and feeders in the backyard? Has the *person* ever visited an aviary?

The Arts: Take pictures of birds splashing in the birdbath.

Exercise: Taking a walk around the bird sanctuary is a good way to incorporate physical activity into the daily routine. Bag the food, fill the feeders, put away the food, and stretch to check on each feeder daily.

Humor: Laugh about birds flocking to the feeder just like people lining up for lunch.

Late Dementia: Make frequent stops by the window to observe the birds. Position the *person's* chair by the window or sit together on a bench outside. Point out the birds.

Old Sayings: "That's for the birds!" "Birds of a feather flock together."

Sensory: Bird sanctuaries provide sounds to hear, such as the chirping of baby birds.

Spirituality: Participating in the care of nature's wonders gives an exhilarating feeling of being part of something greater than yourself.

Conversation: Reminisce, "Did you ever find a nest full of baby birds?" Ask opinions, "What do you think about blue jays?" Give compliments, "You do a great job filling that bird feeder everyday." or "Uriel, did you know that some cultures make Bird's Nest Soup and it's considered quite a delicacy?" Complain, "Those pigeons are awfully greedy. They're eating all the birdseed."

Being in the Community

Many of us have a need to be with others, to get out, to enjoy new places, and to be entertained. Many *persons* with dementia will participate in a variety of activities in the community with a trusted caregiver. The suggestions in this activity will help you employ knack to turn these outings into a special time to observe the world and experience the pleasures of a new adventure.

The Basics

Always be on the lookout for things you can do out of the house. Watch the newspaper for community events and activities, lectures, and concerts. Choose a time of day when the *person* is at his or her best. Some *persons* are best first thing in the morning; others need a few hours to get going and are their best in the afternoon or evening. Plan accordingly.

Following are some ideas for places to go: museums, places of worship, outdoor concerts, library, swimming pool, fitness center, movies, symphony, block parties, grandchildren's activities, sports, parades, park, farmer's market, arboretum, community picnics, and city walking paths.

Tip: Consider attending an adult center. It's highly recommended for *persons* with dementia and gives them a chance to socialize with others (while giving the caregiver a break).

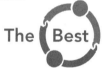

The (Best) Friends Way

Life Story: Tie your activities to the *person's* past interests, such as art museums or garage sales. If the *person* has always enjoyed people, he or she might enjoy going to a community picnic or a sporting event.

The Arts: Take a camera with you as you make your rounds, and take the pictures to create a photo album or bulletin board.

Early Dementia: *Persons* can often help plan the outings.

Exercise: Walking is one of the best exercises, and one that you can adapt to the *person's* pace.

Spirituality: The *person* may enjoy visiting his or her familiar church, synagogue, or mosque; going to a brief music program; or attending a church supper. If the *person* is not a part of a faith community, he or she may find spiritual meaning in taking a walk in the park, visiting a museum, or attending a concert.

Conversation: Comment on an art piece, "Look at all the shades of blue in this painting." Notice the children in the park, "Look at the children playing in the fountain. What a great way to cool off!" Tie to the life story, "We have not missed a Shriner's pancake breakfast for 25 years!" Try to identify trees in the park. Acknowledge the *person*, "Thank you for going places with me."

An ounce of prevention...

Be flexible in your plans. If the person *is becoming overwhelmed, cut the activity short.*

The Basics

Match the *person's* interest, ability, and personality with a pet. Involve the *person* as much as possible with the daily life of the pet (e.g., grooming a dog, feeding exotic fish, changing a bird cage, holding a cat in his or her lap). Being a part of taking the pet to the vet for check-ups and vaccinations can give the *person* a feeling of responsibility.

Tip: If you can't have a pet, visit someone who does or make regular visits to the pet shop or shelter.

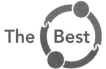

The (Best) Friends Way

Life Story: Has the *person* enjoyed pets before? What type of pet was his or her favorite? Did he or she raise animals on a farm? What kinds of animals has a city *person* been exposed to? *Persons* often have vivid memories of a childhood pet.

The Arts: Create a collage involving pictures and artwork of animals and pets.

Exercise: Take the dog for a walk.

Humor: "That dog eats better than we do!" Laugh at pictures of people and dogs that look alike.

Early Dementia: The *person* can be the primary caretaker of the pet.

Late Dementia: A *person* often enjoys just holding a pet in his or her lap. Sometimes *persons* enjoy pets now even if they did not in the past.

Old Sayings: "A dog is a man's best friend."

Old Skills: Feeding the fish may be something the *person* has done and may remember how to do.

Sensory: A pet provides many hours of tactile stimulation. Enjoy a cat's purr or a dog's soft fur.

Conversation: Reminisce, "I heard that story about when your brother put your doll's dress on a chicken!" Give compliments, "I really admire the way you keep the dog groomed." Demonstrate, "Look, I taught our dog Maggie to shake hands. What do you think about that?"

Caring for Pets

Most pets give unconditional love and can provide us with hours of entertainment. *Persons* with dementia can care for pets and get so much in return.

An ounce of prevention...

Carefully choose a pet when acquiring a new one. Know its history and the characteristics of the breed. Consider getting a retired companion dog that has already been trained or a gentle pet from the animal shelter.

Arranging Fresh Flowers

Everyone enjoys receiving a beautiful bouquet of flowers. It is pleasurable for a *person* with dementia to not only receive flowers, but to actually take part in creating the arrangement! This activity is familiar and has many different levels of accomplishments, making it effective throughout the disease.

The Basics

Choose a variety of fresh-cut flowers to make the arrangement colorful and varied. Take time to look at and smell the flowers. Talk about and name each kind of flower. Decide on a container. Discuss how the flowers should be arranged, how long the stems should be, and how to create the most beautiful flower arrangement. Invite the *person* to place flowers in the container one by one.

Variations: Gathering the flowers could be a separate activity. Enjoy gardening and seed catalogs. Force bulbs to flower in winter. Visit a farmer's market and enjoy seeing all of the variety of flowers for sale direct from the growers.

The 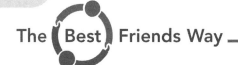 Best Friends Way

Life Story: Has the *person* had a long-held interest in flowers. Did he or she have a beautiful garden? Has the *person* ever visited England to see the beautiful gardens? Find out if the *person* has a favorite flower.

The Arts: Use some of the fresh-cut flowers to inspire a still-life drawing (see page 50), or for flower pounding (see page 66).

Humor: Joke about how men often give women flowers when they're in trouble!

Early Dementia: Ask a *person* who enjoys arranging flowers to create floral arrangements for a church night supper or a family party.

Old Skills: Some *persons* have arranged flowers since they first picked a bunch of daisies as a child.

Sensory: Consider putting fresh herbs such as rosemary or mint into the arrangement. Have the *person* crush the herb with his or her fingertips and enjoy the aroma.

Conversation: Give compliments, "I like the way you put the tall flowers in the middle. Now we can enjoy these short flowers that are so pretty." Spend time admiring the arrangement, "It is so colorful and fragrant." Reminisce with a brother, "When we were young you always bought flowers from the carts in the city? You always brought flowers to Mother." Try to solve a problem together, "I wonder how the flowers get their beautiful colors." Encourage, "You are doing a great job. I want you to continue."

The Basics _____

When planning the trip, assess the *person's* ability to change routine, his or her functional ability, and his or her needs. Plan the appropriate length of the trip as well as the best destination for enjoyment.

Day trips can be a great way to travel without being away from the security of home for too long. If you travel overnight, consider inviting another family member, friend, or paid caregiver to accompany you for additional support. Keep your plans flexible in case you need to come home early.

Traveling

Many people have enjoyed traveling, whether for a day trip or an extended vacation. Other times they have traveled to attend an important family event or business meeting. Modifying the experience of travel can help a *person* with dementia continue to enjoy the experiences of taking a trip.

The  Best Friends Way _____

Life Story: When planning the destination, consider the *person's* favorite places. Visit his hometown, go to the beach if she has always enjoyed it, or visit a historical landmark that the *person* is interested in.

Early Dementia: *Persons* with early dementia may be able to do some extensive traveling and may not be limited to day trips or even staying in the country as long as they are with a caregiver or friend who understands the disease.

Music: Create a ritual of singing the song "On the Road Again" each time you set out for an adventure! Bring the *person's* favorite music along to play during the trip.

Sensory: Traveling has so many things to experience and stimulate the senses: trying a new local food, smelling the saltwater coming off the ocean, feeling the sand between your toes, or smelling a magnolia tree in full bloom.

Spirituality: You may take a trip back to the *person's* roots, attend a religious service, visit a family's mountain retreat, or go to any place that gives a feeling of spiritual renewal.

Conversation: Ask for an opinion, "What do you think it was like to live in a cabin like this in the 1800s?" Reminisce, "Did you ever look for seashells on the beach?" Discuss the best way to travel, "Is it better to drive or to fly?" Remark on nature's beauty, "Aren't the trees here beautiful? You can tell by the colors that fall is here."

An ounce of prevention…

Always think safety! Choose locations that are not too crowded or overwhelming. At a certain point, travel with the person is not advisable…. Utilize Safe Return to provide an extra measure of security.

Using the Computer

Computers play an important role in many homes today, providing games, information, and e-mail to stay in touch with others. Many *persons* with dementia have used a computer in their work and leisure and want to continue with past practices.

The Basics

Assess the *person's* past usage of the computer, and develop a plan to help him or her continue in some way. Sensitive caregivers may need to stand by and serve as a "technological expert" when surprises pop up.

Use the computer together to plan trips, look up family genealogy, research a topic, or play a simple game such as solitaire. Follow an on-line real-life adventure such as web reports from people climbing Mt. Everest or sailing across the Pacific.

The 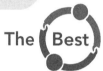 Best Friends Way

Life Story: Know how the *person* used the computer in the past. Was it for work, getting information, or some other use? What is his or her functional level with the computer now?

Humor: Make jokes about losing files on the computer.

Early Dementia: There are a growing number of Internet chat rooms and services for *persons* with early stages of dementia.

Late Dementia: *Persons* may enjoy sitting beside you while you are reading information and looking at pictures on the Internet.

Music: You can play compact discs and listen to songs on the Internet.

Sensory: Many games have sounds and rich visual stimulation with bright colors and movement.

Conversation: Encourage the *person* by sharing your feelings in a humorous way, "Some days I feel like throwing this computer out the window!" Marvel together, "Who ever would have thought that we would be able to send messages to the top of Mt. Fuji?" Compliment, "You have been an old pro at this for a long time." Have fun reminiscing about the journey from manual typewriters, to high-end typewriters, to early word processors, and to the development of the Internet.

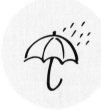

An ounce of prevention...

If the person is comfortable with the computer, try to avoid upgrading or changing anything that the person uses because it may be too difficult to learn something new. Monitor the person's computer usage as you would any activity.

The Basics

There are a surprising number of steps to doing the laundry, including gathering clothes to be washed, sorting clothes, putting clothes in the washer, adding detergent, transferring clothes to the dryer, hanging clothes outside to dry, folding, pressing, ironing, and putting clothes away. Some garments require hand washing.

Try to figure out the most appropriate step or steps for the *person*. Let that be the *person's* specific job. Talk about his or her help in keeping the laundry caught up and how much you appreciate the contribution.

Laundry

Doing the laundry is something everyone has to deal with. Some of us love doing the laundry, and others avoid it if at all possible. For those *persons* with dementia who have always enjoyed being a laundry expert, this activity can be a favorite one.

The 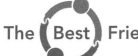 Best Friends Way

Life Story: Many *persons* have been in charge of the laundry all of their lives. Does the *person* seem to have an interest in helping with the laundry now? Did he or she ever work in a laundry or help other individuals with their laundry?

Humor: Laugh together about the time you washed a red sock with all the whites and turned everything pink! Or comment that there are ten socks without a matching one; the washer must be eating the socks!

Early Dementia: *Persons* may be completely functional in a task as familiar as operating the washer and dryer. They may take great pride in washing by hand some of their articles of clothing.

Late Dementia: *Persons* can find meaning in folding clothes, especially bath towels, tea towels, and napkins.

Old Sayings: "Starched stiff enough to stand alone."

Old Skills: Folding, ironing, and hanging clothes out to dry are activities many people conducted all of their lives.

Sensory: The soft feel of fabric and the clean smell of clothes can be wonderfully refreshing. And if hanging clothes outside is the order of the day, the whole outside is a sensory show.

Conversation: Reminisce, "Do you remember your mother using a washboard to clean the clothes?" "Did you hang your clothes out to dry on a line?" Ask for advice, "What is the best way to get out a stain?" Compliment, "Marilyn, you must have worked so hard to send your girls to school in a clean starched dress every day" or "Matt, I can tell you learned how to iron in the Marines. I've never seen neater pants with such a crisp look."

After-Dinner Activities

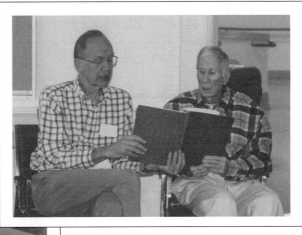

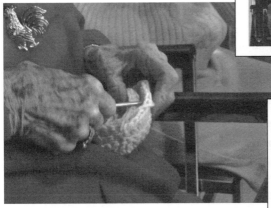

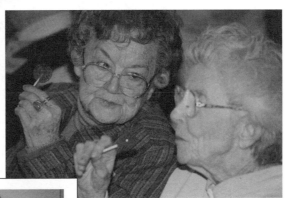

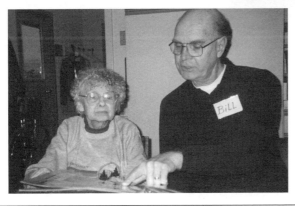

After-Dinner Activities

When we think about our own evenings, the pace may slow down, but we still are doing many things. We may do household chores, watch a movie, go out with friends, read a book, or prepare for a work meeting the next day. *Persons* with dementia share similar desires to stay busy. It is imperative that programs offer activities after dinner, and that staff members also have some tricks up their sleeves for the *person* who gets up at 3 o'clock in the morning and needs some attention.

Instead, after dinner is served, many residential care activity programs come to a full stop. This happens because the activity staff have gone home and because some program managers have (wrongly) argued that the residents are too tired to take part in activities. As a result, some *persons with dementia* become bored, go to bed early, and then wake up during the night. Those who stay up also get bored and can exhibit challenging behaviors or even attempt to wander off during this time.

Compounding these challenges is the impact of dementia on a *person's* sleep cycle. Many *persons* begin to exhibit restlessness and agitation in the later afternoon. Sleep cycles are often affected, and a *person* may be awake during the night and sleep during the day. Dementia may also cause confusion about times and the difference between night and day.

Evening staff should receive training and support to do easy, one-to-one or small group activities with night-owl residents. A staff member with knack who invests 10 minutes with a restless resident can make a profound difference.

Family caregivers can readily adopt the activities in this chapter at home. Caregivers can choose from activities that require their direct involvement, such as *Reading Aloud* (see page 187) or lower energy ones that require minimal supervision, such as *Watching Television* (see page 188) or *Listening to Music* (see page 189).

In residential care settings, a number of activities can be utilized after dinner in small groups. *Postcard Collages* (see page 181), for example, can be worked on in a large group during the day and then be left out for persons who wish to continue working in the evening.

Having an evening activity program in a residential facility supports dignity and happiness by improving quality of life. It is also a mark of quality for a dementia special care program. We believe that even small efforts in this area will pay big dividends.

CHAPTER NINE ACTIVITIES

The Basics

Invite one *person* or a small group to join you on an evening walk-about. The following are some places to invite *persons* to discover: watching the tropical fish in the tank, searching for the resident cat, critiquing the artwork in the halls, examining a map with pegs noting the birthplace of each resident, checking new blooms on the flowers in the sun room, trying out the new furniture in the living room or lounge, watching the birds in the aviary, or studying a bulletin board.

Variation: Make a scavenger hunt out of the activity.

Touring the Inside

Have you ever enjoyed a tour of a friend's new home? It's interesting and fun to explore a new terrain. Residential communities are filled with interesting nooks and corners for *persons* with dementia to explore in the evenings. This activity can be helpful for *persons* who have lots of energy to expend before going to bed or who get up during the night.

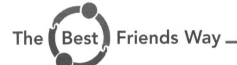

The (Best) Friends Way

Life Story: As you tour, make connections between what you are seeing and the *person's* life. With someone who played the piano, examine the piano as you walk by and see if it's in tune. With someone who enjoyed decorating, look at the décor and discuss if it was done in good taste. When walking with a retired carpenter, comment on the bookshelves, the installation of the ceiling fans, and the quality of the workmanship. This is caregiving knack at its best—engaging a *person* in effective and person-centered conversation.

The Arts: Stop and study the painting in the hallway. Discuss the subject matter, colors, and technique. Admire the gold-leaf frame of the picture. Ask if the painting reminds the *person* of anything.

Exercise: Exploring can be excellent exercise.

Humor: "Who knows? We may even find an ice cream sundae around the corner."

Early Dementia: Invite a *person* who enjoys helping others to push a *person* in a wheelchair, and all three of you tour the inside together.

Sensory: Go by the kitchen and smell the aroma of bread or cookies baking.

Spirituality: Visit the chapel with a *person* who enjoys the serenity and peacefulness of that space.

Conversation: Find the individual in charge of maintenance and encourage the *person* with dementia to walk with him or her and discuss that day's chores and activities. Compliment, "I know you always enjoyed decorating your house. Come with me to see the new furniture in the lounge." Count together, "Let's see how many hibiscus blossoms this plant has today. It's your turn to count!"

Sit Beside Me

What is it like to sit beside someone special? These times provide us all with moments of happiness. Sitting beside a best friend in the evening can be particularly comforting for a *person* with dementia.

The Basics

Brainstorm places to sit beside the *person,* such as at a staff member's desk sorting papers, at the kitchen table peeling potatoes and looking at recipes, in the hallway stealing a few minutes to just talk, or on a screened-in porch on a summer evening.

Remind staff that a brief visit is okay—just spending 3 minutes with someone visiting one-to-one can be meaningful.

Training Tip: Role playing can be a good way to show the benefits of this activity.

The 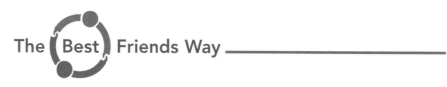 Best Friends Way

Life Story: Look at the *person's* life story for some one-to-one activities or topics to discuss while sitting beside the *person.* Examples include looking at baseball trading cards, talking about the *person's* interest in dog shows, discussing fashion with a former department store saleswoman, reading a hometown newspaper, or playing a hand of cards or game of dominos with someone who enjoyed those activities.

The Arts: Enjoy looking through a book of famous paintings.

Late Dementia: Sit close enough for the *person* to feel the warmth of your body, put your arm around him or her if that feels appropriate, hold hands. Be present for the *person*; being totally present for another is a gift.

Music: Sing a familiar song together.

Sensory: Invite the *person* to relish in the quiet of this moment and to be conscious of the in and out of his or her relaxed breathing.

Spirituality: Read a sacred text, say a prayer together, or listen if the *person* wants to talk about his or her spiritual life.

Conversation: Incorporate humor into the conversation, "We're just like two peas in a pod." Reassure the *person* who is sad and lonely, "I am so glad that the two of us can spend time together." Reminisce, "Wasn't the French Quarter in New Orleans near your home?" or "It's nice to sit next to someone quietly isn't it, Marcel? I know that you enjoyed many quiet times hiking in the Sierra. Tell me about those times."

The Basics _____

- Six postcards (either new postcards or old postcards donated by friends and family)
- Colored posterboard
- White glue
- Scissors
- White construction paper
- Black pen, pencil

Cut white construction paper to a size that will frame each postcard, leaving approximately a 2" border along the bottom (approximately 5" by 7"). With a pencil, trace an outline on the construction paper where the postcard will go.

Find the caption on the back of the postcard that tells about the picture. Copy the caption with a black pen onto the bottom 2" border of the white paper frame.

Glue postcards to the white frames. Arrange the framed postcards onto the colored posterboard. Discuss each postcard. Hang in a strategic place on the wall at eye level to be enjoyed.

Planning Tip: You can prepare the materials in advance and then use them in the evenings with residents.

Variations: Make a postcard album by placing postcards in a small photo album. It is easy to hold and can be looked at anytime. Make a postcard guessing game by gluing postcards onto posterboards without the descriptions. Have the participants guess the places shown on the photos.

Postcard Collages

Postcards bring a smile to all of us, evoking memories of past trips, connections with friends and family, and far-away places. This activity uses postcards to create a colorful collage that can cue meaningful memories of *persons* with dementia.

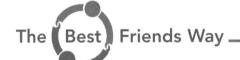

The (Best) Friends Way _____

Life Story: This activity lends itself well to celebrating a *person's* life story. Tie the collage into a hometown, a favorite vacation spot, or a love of nature or animals. Find out if the *person* regularly sent postcards to friends and family when he or she traveled. Did he or she keep an elaborate address book?

Early Dementia: A *person* with early dementia can write the descriptions on the border of each postcard and glue the cards in place.

Humor: Many postcards exemplify "goofy" humor—for example the fictitious animal "the jack-alope" or silly postcards such as a dolphin wearing an "itsy-bitsy-teeny-weeny yellow polka-dot bikini."

Conversation: Ask easy questions, "Does that look like a place you would like to visit?" or "Do people send postcards as much as they used to?" Ask for help, "How long does it take a postcard to get overseas?" Dream, "Here's a postcard of the Eiffel Tower. Would you like to go to the top of it and look out?"

Remember When?

Reflecting on our lives and recalling meaningful moments from the past brings pleasure to many people. Because long-term memories outlast short-term ones for *persons* with dementia, activities that evoke reminiscing tend to be successful.

The Basics

On separate index cards, write statements that begin with, "Remember when…" Utilize books and the Internet for background information. Use photos that relate to the memories. Gather a small group of *persons* to reminisce about each topic. Here are a few suggestions:

- Remember when milk was delivered by a milkman…
- Remember when The Beatles came to America…
- Remember when there were trolley cars…
- Remember when we looked forward to looking through the Sears & Roebuck catalog…
- Remember when there was no color television…
- Remember when John Kennedy was president…
- Remember when man first walked on the Moon…

These cards can be used one-to-one if a *person* wakes up during the night.

The 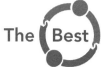 Best Friends Way

Life Story: Use each *person's* Life Story to generate ideas for the "Remember When" topics. For instance, if one *person* in the group loved Elvis, share memories of him.

Humor: Create cards that evoke funny memories, "Remember when you were most embarrassed…"

Early Dementia: Invite *persons* to help you select the "Remember When" topics.

Sensory: Enjoy laughing together. The simple act of laughing can be a powerful experience for our bodies and souls and is healthy, too.

Spirituality: Remembering one's life and looking back on the past provides an opportunity to reflect and celebrate the journey.

Conversation: Let the cards be your guide for your conversation. Ask additional questions to further the discussion such as: "What was that like?" or "Herman, what did you do when that happened?" Reminisce, "How did you feel about it?" Discuss the meaning of the phrase "good old days." Compliment, "Larry, I can't believe that you are old enough to remember that!"

An ounce of prevention…

Be cautious that the memories talked about are not too painful for some persons. *Be sensitive if* persons *seem uncomfortable.*

The Basics _____

- Plain white paper
- Colored pencils or crayons
- Lace scraps

Place a piece of lace under a sheet of paper. Lightly rub a pencil or crayon evenly on the paper. Color a few lace designs on the same page. Try different colors. You may also cut them out and glue them to a card.

Variations: Place the paper over an award, a recognition plaque, and rub crayon over it to pick up the words and design. Paper doilies and leaves can also make interesting rubbings.

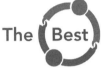

The (Best) Friends Way _____

Life Story: Find out if the *person's* mother or grandmother made lace. Was the *person* interested in sewing or fabrics? Did she have a lace tablecloth to use for formal dinner parties? Did the *person* ever have a lace dress? Does the *person* have a reward plaque that you can make a rubbing of?

Early dementia: A *person* may be able to do tatting, a simple form of lacework.

Music: Ask if anyone can sing the song, "Chantilly Lace."

Old Skills: The activity enhances hand–eye coordination.

Sensory: Have as many different kinds of lace on hand as possible to pass around and stimulate discussion. How does the lace feel?

Spirituality: Discuss christening gowns and why special time and care was taken to make these gowns. Have the gowns been passed from generation to generation? What does that mean to the *person*?

Conversation: Talk about all the things lace can be used for. Reminisce, "Julia, did your mother have lace handkerchiefs? Are they easy to iron?" Ask an opinion, "Mrs. Petersen, do you think this lace would look nice on a wedding dress?" Explore a topic together, "I wonder how they make lace?" Reminisce, "Did you ever do a brass rubbing?"

Lace Rubbings

This activity, in which paper is placed on top of lace and colorful rubbings are created, is good for a quick one-to-one project or for a small group in the evening. It requires few materials and lends itself to a variety of discussion. Lace is rich with memories and symbolic meaning to many *persons* with dementia.

Tea Time

It's tea time! In the evening, tea time can be a soothing activity for a small group or even one-to-one, and herbal teas can encourage sleep. This activity provides *persons* with dementia with stimulating conversation, warm tea, and sweet treats.

The Basics

- Information and trivia about tea. (Internet keywords: herbal remedies, history of tea, tea leaves fortune telling, Earl Grey.)
- Different flavors/varieties of tea (e.g., peach, cinnamon, mint, lemon, Darjeeling, Earl Grey, lapsang souchong, oolong, green tea)
- Teapots, mugs, or china teacups to set around the table
- Cookies or scones

Prepare a dozen trivia questions on cards that can be used by staff whenever they do this activity. Give participants a choice of tea from a box or basket of assorted teas. Serve with a cookie or scone. Discuss tea time and ask the prepared questions. At the end, read everyone's fortune in the tea leaves.

Be sure to encourage *persons* to help with serving. This activity is easy to adapt one-to-one late at night.

The 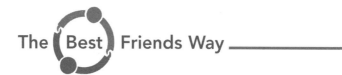 Best Friends Way

Life Story: Make sure you know how a *person* likes his or her tea served (with lemon, milk, sugar, honey, or plain). Did anyone live or travel where tea is grown? Does anyone's tradition include tea time (United Kingdom) or tea ceremonies (Japan)?

Humor: Laugh about holding the tea cup with the little finger sticking out. Joke about reading tea leaves, "I think the leaves at the bottom of your cup suggest a million dollars is coming your way."

Music: Softly sing "Tea for Two" and "I'm a Little Teapot."

Old Sayings: "Not for all the tea in China." "Not my cup of tea." "Tempest in a teapot."

Sensory: Taste and enjoy the rich aroma of the tea and the flavor of the treats. Enjoy the colors and patterns on the teacups and saucers.

Conversation: Discuss a remedy, "Did you ever drink chamomile tea to help you sleep?" Give a choice, "Do you prefer hot tea or iced tea?" Learn together, "What country produces the most tea in the world?" (India) or discuss the Boston Tea Party. "What does the expression 'hot the pot' mean?" (One should heat the teapot with hot water before adding the boiling water to the tea leaves to ensure the hottest pot of tea.)

The Basics

Use vintage photos and pictures from books, magazines, or the Internet. Converse about the subject of the photograph—for example, the occasion caught on film, the general era, or the occupations of the individuals pictured. Look for pictures with good contrast for easier viewing.

Variation: Use family photos or photos taken in your program for discussion. A similar activity can be done with contemporary color photographs.

Vintage Photographs

Photographs are a visual record of the past. They can be of people, famous or unknown, interesting places, or historic events. Photographs can help *persons* with dementia stay connected to their long-term memories. This can be a relaxing one-to-one or small group activity in the evening.

The 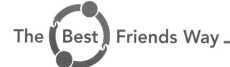 Best Friends Way

Life Story: In gathering the photographs, try to tie them to the actual life experiences of members of the group. For example, someone who was raised in Hawaii may enjoy pictures of beaches and surfers. Someone who lived in Pittsburgh might enjoy looking at pictures of old steel factories.

Humor: Find humor in old hairstyles or period bathing outfits that look like someone is fully dressed compared with today's skimpy swimsuits.

Old Sayings: "A picture is worth a thousand words." "Pretty as a picture."

Sensory: Enjoy looking at the pictures. The contrasts between black and white will be stimulating. Holding the book or the magazine will provide tactile stimulation.

Spirituality: Caregivers with knack enjoy philosophical moments. Explore together the passage of time and the potential impact we have on others, "What will people say about us someday when they look at our picture?"

Conversation: Review close-up portraits and, when it's hard to tell, conduct an entertaining survey, "Is this a man or a woman?" Reminisce, "Do you remember your first portrait?" Speculate, "What do you think is happening in this photo? Do you think he lives in the city or the country?" Share a story, "I think I took better pictures with my old Brownie Box camera than with today's fancy cameras!"

Chewing the Fat

Many of us have enjoyed the camaraderie of sitting with others and just chatting (chewing the fat). Even though caregivers and staff realize that *persons* with dementia lose language skills, talking with one another in the evenings can still be meaningful. This can be a great activity that brings a sense of normalcy back into a *person's* life.

The Basics

Many *persons* are very social and like to visit with others. It becomes more and more difficult, however, for them to initiate conversation.

Invite a few *persons* (two or more) and initiate a basic conversation about weather, sports, tools, anything of interest. Facilitate as needed, but let the group carry on, as much as possible, on their own. For instance, a group could meet at a certain time each week for an hour after dinner. Have snacks available to add to the social aspects of the activity.

The 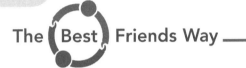 Best Friends Way

Life Story: Bring *persons* together who have similar interests and backgrounds, which will allow for easier conversation. Begin the conversation by drawing from each of their life stories, "Bob did you know that Mark was also a musician?"

Humor: Chewing the fat easily lends itself to telling jokes or funny stories.

Old Sayings: "Chewing the fat." "Shooting the breeze."

Old Skills: The very nature of talking with each other is an old skill.

Sensory: Enjoy laughing together. The simple feel of laughter to our bodies and souls can be a powerful and healthy experience.

Conversation: Clarify, "Thomas, were you and Benjamin both in the Navy?" Notice that Scott has brought something with him, and ask him to show his plaque to everyone. Comment, "That must have been a proud moment when you received this great honor." Encourage stories, "Marvin, James is new and hasn't heard about the time you lost your 400-pound hog off of your truck. Tell him that funny story." Ask an opinion, "Isn't today cool for July?"

An ounce of prevention...

Some persons *will find a natural rapport with one another; others will not. Choose your group wisely.*

The Basics

Build a collection of reading-aloud materials. Choose familiar readings, prayers, poems, and jokes.

Find a place for a small group to meet. It is important to meet in the same place and at the same time. Decide on a name for the group, such as Study Club or Book Club. This can also be an individual activity in the home or a residential setting.

Consider some bedside reading with a *person* to evoke nostalgic memories and help them go to sleep.

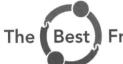

The (Best) Friends Way

Life Story: Take note of those who have an interest in reading of any kind. Have *persons* been teachers, worked in a library, or read to children and grandchildren?

Humor: There are funny joke books, misquotes in newsletters and newspapers, and many humorous poems and stories.

Early Dementia: *Persons* often can read exceedingly well. They should be encouraged to read aloud to the group.

Late Dementia: *Persons* in late dementia can respond to very familiar prayers, readings, and childhood rhymes. They should be encouraged to be a part of the group if they seem to enjoy it.

Music: Reading the lyrics from familiar songs can prompt *persons* to break into song.

Old Skills: Reading aloud is an old skill, fine-tuned through the years, and is often intact far into the disease.

Sensory: The rhythmic tone of being read to can be calming and reassuring.

Spirituality: *Persons* can be connected to their particular religious or spiritual quest by hearing meaningful selections read aloud to them.

Conversation: Celebrate, "We have this nice place for our reading group and lots of interesting material to read." Compliment, "Myrtle, I know you have spent many hours reading stories to be recorded for the blind. That was a wonderful contribution" or "Nellie, I love your reading style." Ask for an opinion, "Mark, I know you taught ancient literature. Did you have a favorite fable?"

Reading Aloud

Many of us have fond memories of being read to as children or reading aloud to our own children. *Persons* with dementia can often read aloud very well even when they are having trouble with conversation.

Watching Television

Most of us enjoy watching television for entertainment and relaxation. With dementia, attention spans shrink, and the ability to understand and interpret stimuli changes. Yet for some caregivers and *persons* with dementia, television programs may be an easy-to-enjoy activity and one particularly suited to the evenings.

The Basics

Carefully choose the type of programs to watch. Short programs work best. Avoid shows with violence and other uncomfortable situations such as extended coverage of breaking news stories. The most successful programs are comedies, game shows, musicals, sports, nature shows, travelogues, and classic movies. Many classic movies and television shows are now on videotape or DVD.

Don't let television-watching dominate your activities. It should be on for purposeful watching, not a constant background.

Variation: In home settings watch old family movies or videotapes.

The 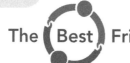 Friends Way

Life Story: Think about the programs the *person* liked best when he or she was younger, possibly "Andy Griffith," "Lawrence Welk," or "I Love Lucy." What interests does the *person* have that could be fulfilled by a television program (e.g., history, sports, dog shows, home improvement)?

Early Dementia: If the *person* enjoys movies, gradually adapt to changes in memory by choosing light, positive movies. If needed, provide gentle reminders of who the characters are and what has already happened.

Humor: Laugh at humorous scenes, such as a talking horse or a dog dressed in fancy clothes.

Music: Television has many musical shows that the *person* may enjoy.

Sensory: Sometimes a calming, soothing video can be added to the *person's* daily routine, especially at bedtime.

Spirituality: A *person* may enjoy watching selected pieces of televised religious services or other programs related to art, music, or nature.

Conversation: Seek an opinion, "What do you think of that?" Say in a humorous tone, "You never know what they will come up with next!" Recall a time when there were just three networks and public television! Exclaim, "Charlotte, those ice skaters are amazing. I enjoyed watching them, did you?" Have fun reminiscing about early television and the purchase of your first color TV.

An ounce of prevention...

Problems of perception may lead the person *to believe that the characters are real or that something they saw on television has happened to a loved one.*

The Basics _____

Listen to music together. Use music that has a positive effect on the *person*. Watch the *person's* body language for cues about whether he or she is enjoying the music. Is there a smile? Does the body sway? Are the eyes closed? Is he or she singing the lyrics to the song?

Variations: Nature sounds such as a bubbling brook, the wind, and the ocean are often available on CD or cassette tape. Usually *persons* enjoy hearing the music they've always loved, but also try something new. Be creative; try a "night at the opera." Dress up as if going to an opera, listen to a favorite opera, enjoy refreshments afterward, and celebrate an entertaining evening.

Listening to Music

Music is something almost all of us have enjoyed throughout our lives. It can evoke laughter or tears and remind us of particular periods in our life. Music fills a void for *persons* with dementia when spoken words and language begin to fail. Though listening to music can be appropriate anytime, it is a very easy activity for the evening.

The 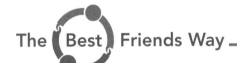 Friends Way _____

Life Story: Know his or her preferred music. Is it country and western, opera, gospel, or jazz? Some songs evoke feelings or memories about the past, such as songs popular during the *person's* teenage years. Did the *person* attend a memorable concert or opera? A Broadway show? A Las Vegas revue?

Exercise: Dance to the music.

Late Dementia: *Persons* in late dementia can relate to music long after they have lost most of their ability to verbally communicate. Look for slight responses to signify enjoyment.

Old Sayings: "That is music to my ears!" "It isn't over 'til the fat lady sings."

Old Skills: Listening to music is an old skill that has been fine-tuned through the years.

Spirituality: Religious music can help some *persons* stay connected to their faith. Others may find that a wonderful opera nurtures the spirit.

Conversation: Ask an opinion, "Do you like the music of Frank Sinatra?" Reminisce, "Do you and your wife have a special song?" Be armchair critics, "How do you think this opera singer compares to others? Is she hitting all the high notes?" Share an opinion, "I like big band music. What about you?" Compliment, "I like the same kind of salsa music you do. We have great taste, don't we?"

Wrapping Presents

Wrapping presents is an old skill that involves planning, decision making, and some physical dexterity. *Persons* with dementia can participate in part or all of the activity. It makes for a mellow but pleasurable evening activity.

The Basics

- Presents to wrap
- Wrapping paper (see Creating Wrapping Paper, page 80)
- Clear tape
- Ribbon
- Gift sacks and colorful tissue paper

This activity can include a small group or a single *person*. Look for occasions when gift wrapping may be needed, including birthdays, holidays, prizes, or thank-you gifts. Gift sacks and colorful tissue are easier than wrapping paper for some *persons* to use. The activity should be relaxed with time to talk about the gifts.

Variation: Staff can bring in presents they intend to give to friends and family members and ask *persons* for help wrapping them.

The 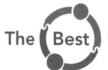 Best Friends Way

Life Story: Who likes to keep their hands busy? Does a *person* enjoy the company of others when they are all working together? Was he or she the one in the family who always wrapped the presents for every occasion?

The Arts: Packages can be very artfully wrapped and decorated. Encourage creativity.

Humor: Keep the conversation light and tease about getting a job as a full-time gift wrapper or quip about sending some of the gifts to yourself.

Early Dementia: This is a satisfying activity for *persons* with early dementia who can tackle wrapping presents on their own.

Late Dementia: Don't forget *persons* in late dementia in this activity. They can help in some small way such as holding the ribbon or tape for you.

Sensory: The bright colors of the paper, rustling of the tissue paper, handling of the gifts, and hubbub of the occasion all engage the senses.

Conversation: Reminisce, "Lucy, I'll bet that you were the one in your family to wrap all the presents." Ask for an opinion, "Would you use this color ribbon with this paper?" Try to figure out, "James, look at this thing. What on earth is it?" Share feelings, "I like to stay busy. Have you always liked to keep busy, too?" Ask for help, "Would you hold your finger right here so I can tie this bow. Thanks, that is just what I needed."

The Basics ─────────────

Create your own, large-type songbooks with lyrics from familiar songs. It's always best to look for a volunteer or staff member to be a pianist, guitarist, or other musical accompanist, but sing-along tapes are available.

Be consistent. Meet in the same location at the same time (just after dinner if possible), and have a defined length of time for singing, such as 30 minutes. Decide on a name for the group such as "The Song Birds." Arrange the seating in a semicircle around the accompanist. It is fun to have a theme song to begin and a favorite song for the ending. Enjoy hymns or religious music now and then, but be sensitive to persons who come from different backgrounds. This activity can be done any time, but for nighttime, slow down the pace.

Sing-Along

Human beings are made to sing. *Persons* with dementia can recall the words of familiar songs and delight in having an opportunity to sing, making this a favorite evening activity.

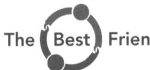

The (Best) Friends Way ─────────────

Life Story: Did anyone sing together as a family around the piano when they were growing up? Are there choir members from hometown churches, communities, or schools? Was anyone a professional singer? Who sang in the shower?

The Arts: Change the names in some songs to include members of the group, such as changing the name in "Good Night Irene" to Matthew or Corrine. Write new verses to some songs.

Exercise: Singing is good for deep breathing and is relaxing at the end of the day.

Humor: Talk and laugh about not being able to carry a tune. Sing some funny songs and keep the sing-along light hearted and fun.

Early Dementia: *Persons* may be able to play the piano or guitar, call out the number of the page of each song, or lead the singing.

Old Skills: Singing is an old skill, and even those who are nonverbal in conversation can often sing every word to a familiar song.

Sensory: Hearing the tones, feeling the rhythm, and seeing the facial expressions of the singers all excite the senses.

Conversation: Use the life story, "Lottie, let's sing your favorite song, 'Let Me Call You Sweetheart.' I like that one too." Compliment, "Mark, I like to sing next to you. You help me stay in tune." Reminisce, "Did your mother sing songs to you at bedtime when you were a little boy?" Ponder after singing the song, "What is a tootsie wootsie?"

Late-Night Snack

There is something wonderful about a late-night snack. It's a guilty pleasure. When *persons* with dementia stay up late or get up during the night, sometimes a small snack (including one shared by the caregiver) can become a focal point of an activity and provide a comforting feel of home.

The Basics

Have ingredients on hand to prepare snacks, including fruit, cookies, peanut butter and crackers, soups, and sandwiches. Appropriate beverages include herbal teas or milk.

As you make a snack together, remind the person of elements from his or her past, discuss favorite foods, or joke about diets.

The 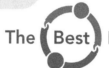 Best Friends Way

Life Story: Did the *person* have a night job or work a late night shift and is accustomed to eating late? Was the *person* a big eater or instead ate small meals throughout the day?

Humor: Joke that you will start your diets tomorrow!

Early Dementia: When the hustle and bustle of the day is over and things quiet down is the time when some of us want to talk. *Persons* in early dementia may use a late-night snack time to talk about what is bothering them.

Late Dementia: *Persons* in late dementia may be hungry but unable to communicate this. If a *person* seems restless, a snack may be the answer.

Music: Put on a favorite song to listen to as background music or even sing a song together.

Spirituality: Some *persons* may find that a prayer or meditation before the snack is comforting and ties into past religious traditions.

Conversation: Ask for advice, "Is this tea strong enough, or does it need to steep longer?" Share traditions, "I always had some warm milk to help me sleep, did you?" Create together, "Let's share a sandwich. What combination is good—turkey and Swiss cheese or ham and Swiss cheese?" Share your feelings, "I'm hungry, what about you?"

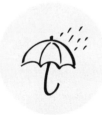

An ounce of prevention...

Tie in choices to a person's dietary needs/requirements. Avoid caffeine and too much sugar late at night.

The Basics

Brainstorm topics that may interest *persons* up late at night such as rereading the newspaper; playing solitaire, table games, and puzzles; or listening to music. A night owl can also "make the rounds" with staff.

Variation: Arrange to have a room open in the evening from the close of dinner to around 9:00 P.M. The regular activity room would be preferred if it is readily accessible. The space can be supervised by a staff member or volunteer. Arrange some chairs for visiting or just watching. Be sure that comfortable seating is offered. Things to do in the gathering room might include: finishing an art project, playing checkers, or looking through theme boxes.

The 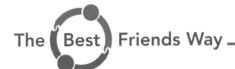 Best Friends Way

Life Story: You may find that some *persons* grew up in families where there were always activities in the evening for family participation. Did the *person* work at night?

The Arts: An activity can be pulled from the chapter called Let's Create. Paint a picture, create a poem, or dance to the music.

Exercise: A small, indoor putting strip might be great exercise for an avid golfer.

Humor: Have funny books or tapes of radio comedy available.

Late Dementia: We often forget that *persons* who no longer choose to actively participate may gain much from being present and watching and listening to all the sights and sounds.

Sensory: Many things in the room can be sensory appealing—the aroma of the fresh flowers waiting to be arranged, the sound of a favorite jazz tune in the background, or the softness of the fabric as a *person* sorts through quilting squares. Herbal teas may facilitate sleep and provide a pleasurable sensory experience.

Spirituality: A *person* might like to hear a favorite religious reading, chat about his or her religious background, or quietly look through a Bible.

Conversation: Ask for help, "Zerelda, would you help me arrange these flowers? Our florist friend sent these cut flowers for us to enjoy." Enjoy looking through the paper together, "I always waited until the end of the day to read the paper. There are so many other things to do during the day. George, would you like to take a look with me?" or "Would you teach me how to play solitaire? I have never played that game in my whole life."

Night Owls

The old saying "early to bed and early to rise" certainly applies to many individuals. However, many *persons* with dementia are "night owls." Creating a special evening room or space with things to do that can keep a *person* occupied but not overstimulated can save the day—or in this case, save the night.

An ounce of prevention...

Supervision is very important for persons who have difficulty initiating an activity. Don't leave persons unattended even though they seem to be occupied.

Mona Lisa and the Art of Good Alzheimer's Care

Here is a challenge we'd like to leave you with as you consider your activity programming or daily activities with *persons* with dementia. Take your current top-five activities and put them on hiatus or "leave" for a month. Challenge yourself—what new activities can you come up with to fill the gap?

Utilize this book for inspiration. Pick five new activities from the book and assemble a brainstorming group to map out how best to conduct these activities in your setting. Have fun, be creative, and don't worry about being "failure free." Remember a key principle of Best Friends activities—the art is not what you do, it is in the doing!

One residential care facility decided to stop playing Bingo for a month in their dementia unit. Bingo was by far the most popular activity, and this decision left some staff members disgruntled. Most of the *persons* with dementia, however, did not notice that Bingo had been stopped.

Bingo was popular because it was fun, easy to do, and involved friendly competition and prizes. Many residents playing Bingo felt successful and engaged. Unfortunately, though, staff members were bored with the game, and their boredom was making the activity stale. Also, staff admitted that the game provided few, if any, opportunities to practice the Best Friends approach to Alzheimer's care, such as reminiscence.

An idea was born to do an activity around the arts, and a classroom atmosphere was created where a famous painting or photograph was shown and discussed. Norman Rockwell prints of nostalgic, small-town American life evoked laughter and memories. Photographs evoked discussions about an individual's hairstyle or clothing, and in one case the famous painting of the Mona Lisa involved the following

- Recognition of the painting as a well-known image
- Sharing of information and trivia about the painting from research on the Internet and an art book
- A chance to spell out the name of the artist, Leonardo da Vinci
- Discussion of Mona Lisa's famous smile (Was she flirting with the artist? Did someone tell a funny joke?)
- Sharing stories of past vacations to Paris, France
- A humorous discussion of Mona Lisa's style (Is she pretty as is or does she need some make-up and jewelry?)
- A chance to play the famous Mona Lisa song, sung by Nat King Cole
- A funny look at Mona Lisa take-offs based on some Internet research
- A chance to draw personal versions of the painting

The afternoon spent on Mona Lisa was wonderful, with laughter, smiles, and fascinating discussion. After the activity, one resident remarked to another, "That was different." The other resident said, "Yes, it was very refreshing." Bingo has its place, but we hope that you will be inspired by the Mona Lisa to refresh your activity program, refresh the *persons* in your care, and refresh yourself the Best Friends way.

Resources for Activities Professionals

Suggested Books

Alzheimer's Association. (1995). *Activity programming for persons with dementia: A sourcebook.* Chicago: Author.

Bell, V., & Troxel, D. (1996). *The best friends approach to Alzheimer's care.* Baltimore: Health Professions Press.

Bell, V., & Troxel, D. (2001). *The best friends staff: Building a culture of care in Alzheimer's programs.* Baltimore: Health Professions Press.

Bell V., & Troxel D. (2002). *A dignified life: The best friends approach to Alzheimer's care.* Deerfield Beach, FL: Health Communications, Inc.

Barrick, A.L., Rader, J., & Hoeffer, B. (2001). *Bathing without a battle: Personal care of individuals with dementia.* New York: Spring Publishing Company.

Basting, A.D., & Killick, J. (2003). *The arts and dementia care: A resource guide.* Brooklyn, NY: The National Center for Creative Aging.

Burdick, L. (2004). *The sunshine on my face.* Baltimore: Health Professions Press.

Chavin, M. (1991). *The last chord: Reaching the person with dementia through the power of music.* Mt. Airy, MD: Eldersong Publications.

Dowling, J.R. (1995). *Keeping busy: A handbook of activities for persons with dementia.* Baltimore: John Hopkins University Press.

Gibson, F. (2004). *The past in the present: Using reminiscence in health and social care.* Baltimore: Health Professions Press.

Hellen, C. (1998). *Alzheimer's disease: Activity focused care.* Boston: Butterworth-Heinemann.

Jenny, S., & Oropeza, M. (1993). *Memories in the making: A program of creative art expression for Alzheimer's patients.* Irvine, CA: Phoenix Press.

Merriam-Webster. (1999). *Merriam-Webster's rhyming dictionary.* New York: Author.

Sheridan, C. (1991). *Reminisce: Uncovering a lifetime of memories.* San Francisco: Elder Press.

Thews, V., Reaves, A.M., & Henry, R.S. (1993) *Now what? A handbook of activities for adult day programs.* Winston-Salem, NC: Bowman Gray School of Medicine at Wake Forest University.

Volicer, L., & Bloom-Charette, L. (1999). *Enhancing the quality of life in advanced dementia.* Philadelphia: Brunner/Mazel.

Wells, S. (1998). *Horticultural therapy and the older adult population.* Binghampton. NY: Haworth Press.

Zgola, J., & Bordillon, G. (2001). *Bon appetit! The joy of dining in long-term care.* Baltimore: Health Professions Press.

Journals

Activity Directors' Quarterly for Alzheimer's & Other Dementia Patients
http://www.alzheimersjournal.com
Editor-in-Chief: Carol F. Lippa

American Journal of Recreation Therapy
http://www.pnpco.com/pn10000.html
Editor-in-Chief: Candace Ashton-Shaeffer

Creative Forecasting
http://www.creativeforecasting.com

Newsletters

Activity Director's Guide and *Here's Help*
Eymann Pulications, Inc.
Post Office Box 3577
Reno, NV 89505
http://www.care4elders.com

Web Sites

Alternative Solutions in Long Term Care
http://www.activitytherapy.com
This web site is a helpful gateway for activity professionals with a rich listing of resource materials,
    holidays, bulletin board ideas, and other materials.

American Horticultural Therapy Association
http://www.ahta.org
This web site is for those interested in the therapeutic benefits of gardening; it includes publica-
    tions and research as well as upcoming events and meetings.

National Alzheimer's Association
http://www.alz.org
This web site contains helpful information for families and professionals coping with Alzheimer's.
    A helpful link to the Greenfield Library contains information for activities professionals.

National Center for Creative Aging
http://www.creativeaging.org/who.html
This is the web site for an organization and a clearinghouse for professionals interested in creativ-
    ity and aging.

The Therapeutic Recreation Director
http://www.recreationtherapy.com
This web site contains resources for recreation therapists, therapeutic recreation specialists, cre-
    ative arts therapists, activity therapists, activity directors, and professionals in other disciplines.

Associations

National Association of Activity Professionals

http://www.thenaap.com

A national group that represents activity professionals.

National Coalition of Creative Arts Therapies Associations (NCCATA)

http://www.nccata.com

An alliance of professional associations dedicated to the advancement of the arts in therapeutic settings.

Establish mutual respect, show understanding, provide support,
and develop the "knack" for being a friend to a person with Alzheimer's disease.

The following examples from *The Best Friends Approach to Alzheimer's Care*
and *The Best Friends Staff* show how even small gestures can be meaningful to a person with dementia.

30 Activities that Can Be Done in 30 Seconds or Less

Greeting the *person* by name

Making eye contact and smiling

Shaking hands

Asking someone to "show me" an object

Teasing, "Mr. Smith, I just saw you eat dessert first!"

Telling someone he or she is loved

Giving a sustained bear hug

Giving a compliment, "Wow! You're looking pretty spiffy today, Margie."

Asking an open-ended question, "How are you feeling today, Mike?"

Asking an opinion, "What do you think of my new necktie? Does it match my shirt?"

Playing a quick game of catch

Noticing an unusual bird out the window

Evoking a memory from the life story of the *person*, "Tell me more about that grandfather of yours who was a country doctor. Did he really make house calls?"

Giving a hand massage

Sharing a new hand lotion and talking about its pleasing scent

Blowing bubbles

Slipping a little treat to someone (being certain it's dietetically okay)

Sharing a magic trick

Showing off family photos of a new grandchild

Blowing up a balloon and batting it around

Looking at a flower arrangement and comparing colors, textures, and scents

Asking for advice on a recipe

Telling a funny story or joke

Doing a quick dance to some fun music playing in the background

Noticing vivid colors in an unusual dress or shirt

Asking for help with a chore, such as folding a towel, helping make a bed, or squirting some wax onto a piece of furniture about to be polished

Trying on a hat or hats

Testing a new shade of lipstick

Clowning around for a moment, making funny faces, or throwing your hands in the air and spinning around once or twice in a silly dance

Stepping outdoors for some fresh air

Expand your knowledge of the Best Friends method with additional titles from Health Professions Press